**Gustavo Correia Basto da Silva
e colaboradores**

DENTAL ANATOMY APPLIED TO DENTAL PRACTICE

Gustavo Correia Basto da Silva
e colaboradores

DENTAL ANATOMY APPLIED TO DENTAL PRACTICE

a study of the permanent and deciduous dentitions

ScienciaScripts

Imprint

Any brand names and product names mentioned in this book are subject to trademark, brand or patent protection and are trademarks or registered trademarks of their respective holders. The use of brand names, product names, common names, trade names, product descriptions etc. even without a particular marking in this work is in no way to be construed to mean that such names may be regarded as unrestricted in respect of trademark and brand protection legislation and could thus be used by anyone.

Cover image: www.ingimage.com

This book is a translation from the original published under ISBN 978-620-4-19274-1.

Publisher:
Sciencia Scripts
is a trademark of
Dodo Books Indian Ocean Ltd., member of the OmniScriptum S.R.L Publishing group
str. A.Russo 15, of. 61, Chisinau-2068, Republic of Moldova Europe
Printed at: see last page
ISBN: 978-620-4-04679-2

Gustavo Correia Basto da Silva

and collaborators

**DENTAL ANATOMY APPLIED TO THE ODENTAL CLINIC: a study of the
permanent and deciduous dentitions**

AUTHOR

GUSTAVO CORREIA BASTO DA SILVA

- Dental Surgeon - UEPB

- Specialist in Collective Health - UFBA

- Specialist in Micropolitics of Management and Work in Health - UFF

- Master in Public Health - UEPB

- Doctoral student in Dentistry - UEPB

- Professor of the Dentistry course - UEPB, Campus VIII

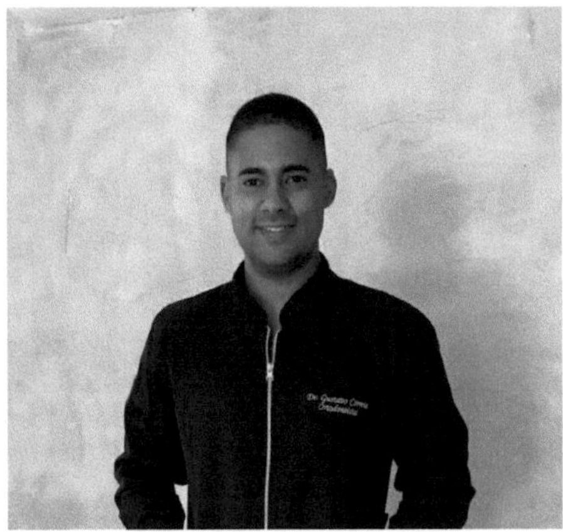

COAUTORS

Suzie Clara da Silva Marques Sabryna Maria Guilhermino Souza Amanda de Almeida Prazeres Moreira Lanna Lidia Monteiro Figueiredo Rayssa de Oliveira Mousinho
Vivian Luana Andrade dos Santos Rebeka Maria de Sousa Feitosa Matheus Andrade Rodrigues Valéria Larissa Costa Oliveira Beatriz Simone Monteiro de Melo Daniela Vasconcelos Silva
Maria Luysa Almeida da Silva Allane Rafaella da Silva Quirino
Yasmim Christynne Oliveira Reis de Freitas Roger Gabriel Karpowicz Menezes
Bruna da Vera Cruz Guedes Camila Moura Maia Dornelas Camila Ketlly Duarte Marinho David Bezerra dos Santos Filho Maria Ismaela Lima de Barros Dias Patrícia Silva Ferreira
Lucas Rodrigues dos Santos Amanda Nandyala Menezes Pinheiro Caroline Belisio Leite de Melo

Joycy Pamella Silva Epifanio Kelly Oliveira da Silva
Lucas Vinicius Viana Machado de Santana Rafaella Soares de Almeida
Edlane da Silva Sousa

Priscylla Gabrielly Brasileiro de Melo Jhulie Lorrany Mendes de Almeida João Paulo Soares de Oliveira Myllenna dos Santos Ferreira
Undergraduates of the Dentistry course - UEPB, campus VIII

PREFACE

The area of Anatomy has been increasingly consolidating in the field of science, as well as holds the power to support decision-making in various clinical and surgical areas. In Dentistry, specifically, the Applied Anatomy is focused on the study of teeth and their correlation with the supporting structures.

Without a thorough anatomical detailing of the dental structure, the undergraduate student in Dentistry - or even the technical courses in the area - will inevitably deal with numerous difficulties in areas where dental sculpture is a prerequisite, since the reproducibility of anatomical accidents in professional practice is key to a good clinical procedure.

In view of this, this book brings to the reader an enlightening approach to the main topics related to Dental Anatomy, both encompassing the groups of permanent teeth and some considerations about the deciduous teeth. Therefore, this work has great potential to provide a thorough study and based on the literature on various topics of Dental Anatomy.

Enjoy your reading!

Prof. Gustavo Correia Basto da Silva

SUMMARY

CHAPTER 1 - PERMANENT INCISORS: A MORPHOLOGICAL APPROACH

Suzie Clara da Silva Marques Sabryna Maria Guilhermino Souza Amanda de Almeida Prazeres Moreira Lanna Lidia Monteiro Figueiredo Rayssa de Oliveira Mousinho
Vivian Luana Andrade dos Santos Rebeka Maria de Sousa Feitosa Matheus Andrade Rodrigues Gustavo Correia Basto da Silva
UPPER CENTRAL INCISOR (11) (21)

GENERALITIES

The upper central incisor is very important in facial aesthetics, since it is located in the most mesial part of the arch and is also essential for speech (MADEIRA, 2004). It occludes with its lower homonym and the mesial part of the lower lateral incisor, being the first tooth of each hemi-arch (Fig **1**) (TEXEIRA, 2001).

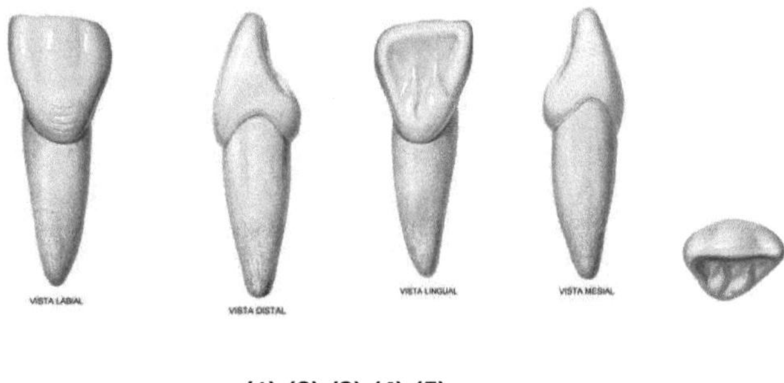

(1) (2) (3) (4) (5)

Figure 1 - Anatomy of the right maxillary central incisor (11). **1** - Buccal face; **2** - Lingual face; **3** - Mesial face; **4** - Distal face; **5** - Incisal edge.

CROWN

VESTIBULAR SIDE

The buccal surface converges cervically through the mesial and distal edges, forming a wider incisal edge. This face is convex and more pronounced in the distal edge, this convexity in the mesiodistal direction is interrupted by the presence of two longitudinal grooves that show the separation of what would be the three developmental lobes. The angle disto-incisal is more rounded than the mesio-incisal, which explains the location of its contact area more cervical (MADEIRA, 2004).

LINGUAL FACE

The mesial and distal faces converge to lingual, and this results in a narrower face compared to the vestibular. It has a concave-convex configuration due to the presence of a fourth developmental lobe called dental cingulum or tubercle, which is a rounded protrusion (TEXEIRA, 2001).

Near the cingulum, a depression, the central fossa, can be observed, which is delimited by marginal ridges that extend laterally from the dental tubercle (TEXEIRA, 2001).

The marginal ridges delimit the central fossa, and as they approach the mesioincisal and distoincisal angles they become less prominent, that is, the depth of the fossa decreases as a result of the lesser thickness of the ridges. Besides these accidents can be observed the presence of tongues, which are protrusions that can mask or even divide the central fossa (TEXEIRA, 2001).

PROXIMAL FACES

The proximal surfaces of the maxillary central incisor are convex along its entire length, however, the mesial surface is less convex and larger in relation to the distal one. The buccal and lingual surfaces converge towards the incisal, providing a similarity with the shape of a triangle. The neck line has its concavity turned towards the root (MADEIRA, 2004)

INCISAL BORDER

When erupting, it is serrated and has three mamelons that with time are worn, in bevel shape, forming a rectilinear surface. This edge is inclined to mesial-distal and cervical because there is a difference in length between the medial and distal face (TEXEIRA, 2001).

COLO

In cross-section, the neck of the maxillary central incisor has a trapezoidal shape with the largest side towards vestibular and the smallest towards lingual. The cervical line is sinuous with smooth concavity towards the crown on the free surfaces and more acute towards the root on the proximal surfaces (TEXEIRA, 2001).

ROOT

The maxillary central incisor is a unirooted tooth, with no bifurcations. (TEXEIRA, 2001) The root is roughly conical in shape and triangular in cross-section. It is wider in the buccal region and narrower in the lingual region and longer than the crown. Its apex is rounded and generally there are no significant distal deviations. (WOOD, 2004)

ERUPTION

The eruption occurs around 7 to 9 years of age and its complete rhizogenesis occurs around 11 years of age (TEXEIRA, 2001).

LOWER CENTRAL INCISOR

GENERALITIES

The incisor teeth are located in the mesial portion of the lower arch of the oral cavity. It is the smallest and most symmetrical tooth of the human permanent dentition. The occlusion is established with the two mesial thirds of the lower central incisor (Fig. **1**) (MADEIRA, 2004).

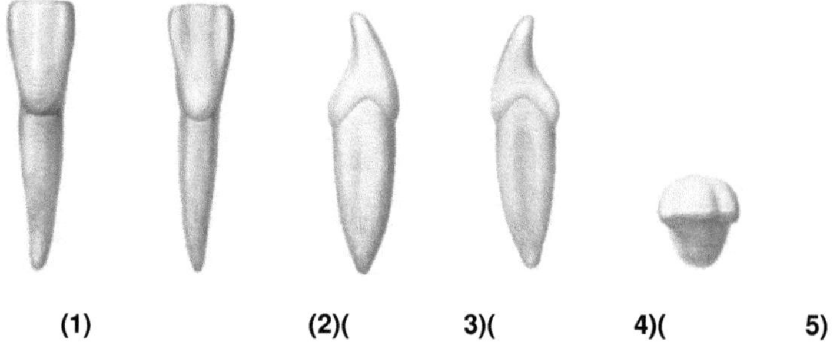

Figure 2 - Anatomy of the right maxillary central incisor (11). **1** - Buccal face;
2 - Lingual face; **3** - Mesial face; **4** - Distal face; **5** - Incisal edge.

CROWN

VESTIBULAR SIDE

It has similarities with the upper central incisors is convex in direction, the mesial sides is larger and longer than the distal the others are quite similar, both are convergent and convex to the neck. The wear on the incisal edges causes the inclination of this to mesial causing greater wear near the mesio-incisal angle.

LINGUAL FACE

It is smaller than the buccal side, is considered a slightly concave face, in the proximal are convergent to the neck having a triangular appearance in it does not present the blind foramen and its marginal ridges are not very visible becoming only be with simple depression.

PROXIMAL FACES

The mesial and distal faces are triangular, with the base facing cervically. They are flat in the cervical and middle thirds and more convex in the incisal third. (MADEIRA, 2004) Both faces are symmetrical, presenting asymmetry when there is wear, which makes one side larger than the other (TEIXEIRA, 2001).

INCISAL BORDER

The incisal edge presents a serrated aspect when the tooth is newly erupted due to the three mamelons. However, as in the maxillary central incisors, masticatory wear makes it rectilinear. In a vestibular view, it has a horizontal format due to the high symmetry of this dental element (TEIXEIRA, 2001).

This edge is displaced lingually in relation to the long axis of the tooth, causing the two incisal thirds of the crown to incline lingually in relation to the root (MADEIRA, 2004).

COLO

In cross-section, has an oval shape with significant flattening in the mesio-distal direction. The cervical line presents as a concavity towards the crown on the free surfaces; on the proximal surfaces, this concavity is more open and turned towards the root (TEIXEIRA, 2001).

ROOT

The inferior central incisor is unirradiculated, without bifurcations. The root is very flat in the mesio-distal direction which makes it elongated in the buccolingual direction with marked longitudinal grooves - especially the distal one (MADEIRA, 2004).

The crown is well centered in relation to the root, highlighting the characteristic of greater symmetry of this tooth. Generally presents little or no deviation; its apex may incline slightly to the vestibular or distal. In cross-section, it is oval-shaped (TEIXEIRA, 2001).

ERUPTION

Their eruption starts around 6 years of age and their complete rhizogenesis occurs between 9 and 10 years of age (TEIXEIRA, 2001).

UPPER LATERAL INCISOR (12) (22) GENERAL

The upper lateral incisor is the second tooth of an upper hemi-arch and its location is between the upper central incisor and upper canine, also receives the name of upper distal incisor (TEXEIRA, 2001). Its shape is similar to the central incisor, but its dimensions are smaller, except the root, has a more variable form than the other teeth and these variations can be considered developmental anomalies such as: pointed shape of the crown, presence of pointed tubercles as part of the cingulum, deep lingual groove covering cingulum and part of the root, crowns and twisted roots, and other malformations (MADEIRA, 2004).

It presents total length of 22.0 mm, being 10.0 mm smaller than the length of the maxillary central incisor, because the mesio-distal diameter is much smaller in the lateral incisor, consequently, the tooth becomes thinner and narrower and with a longer appearance (TEXEIRA, 2001).

The maxillary lateral incisor is the second tooth of each hemi-arch, with its eruption time at 8 years of age, located distally to the maxillary central incisor and mesially to the maxillary canine, having its dimensions reduced in relation to the maxillary central incisor, except for the root length. (TEXEIRA, 2001). There are wide variations in its anatomy as the pointed format in the crown, existence of the pointed tubercle as part of the cingulum, deep lingual groove, twisted roots and crowns, which are considered anomalies (MADEIRA, 2004). (Fig. 3).

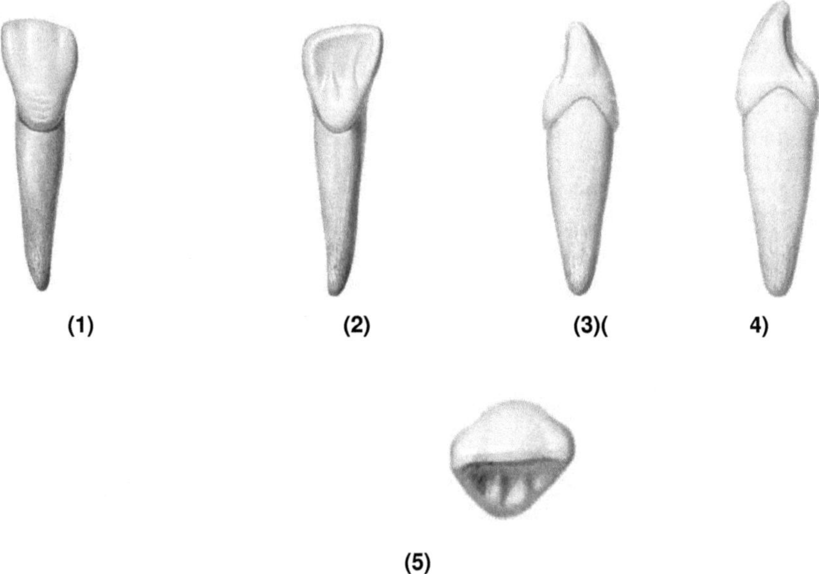

Figure **3 -** Anatomy of upper right permanent lateral incisor: **1-** Buccal face; 2- Palatal face; 3- Mesial face; **4-** Distal face; **5-** Incisal edge

CROWN

VESTIBULAR SIDE

It has a trapezoidal shape, with dimensions in the incisal-cervical direction greater than mesial-distal, it is notable a greater convexity of the face in the cervical third due to the presence of the buccal boss and flat features in the other incisal thirds (TEXEIRA, 2001). The characteristic of the crown is to have its convexity accentuated in the mesial-distal direction where it is limited by the mesial and distal edge, with mesial and disto-incisal angles (MADEIRA, 2004).

PALATINE FACE

The palatal surface is smaller than the buccal surface, characterized by prominences such as the well-developed cingulum and the mesial and distal marginal ridges that are thicker near the cingulum (TEXEIRA, 2001). These three prominences (cingulum, marginal ridge and distal ridge) delimit the lingual fossa, which has a deeper form because of its narrower dimensions. It is worth mentioning the presence of the blind foramen, which is located between the cingulum and lingual fossa (MADEIRA, 2004).

PROXIMAL FACES

They present similarities with the contact faces of the central incisor where the mesial face is larger and has less convexity than the distal. In the cervical third are flat in order to maintain the interdental space and in the incisal third are convex in order to maintain contact (TEXEIRA, 2001).

INCISAL BORDER

The mesial segment is smaller and less inclined, while the distal segment is larger and more inclined, resulting in an accentuated rounding of the distal angle (TEXEIRA, 2001).

COLO

In a cross-section, the upper lateral incisor has an oval shape and the cervical line has the same anatomical aspects of the central incisor, characterizing more closed concavities (TEXEIRA, 2001).

ROOT

The upper lateral incisor is a unirooted tooth with no ramifications. The root has a conical-pyramidal shape, being more tapered and flattened in the mesiodistal direction (TEXEIRA, 2001). Large longitudinal grooves can be seen on the mesial and distal surfaces. And its apical third is more distally deviated (MADEIRA, 2004).

ERUPTION

The eruption of the upper lateral incisors occurs around 8 years of age, being 10 to 12 months the beginning of calcification, from 4 to 5 years the amelogenesis complete and rhizogenesis complete at 11 years. Its occlusion is with the distal half of the lower lateral incisor and the mesial half of the lower canine (TEXEIRA, 2001).

LOWER LATERAL INCISOR (32) (42) GENERAL

The Lower Lateral Incisor is the second tooth of a lower hemiarchus and its location is between the lower central incisor and the lower canine (TEXEIRA). Its shape is similar to the lower central incisor (MADEIRA, 2004), but its crown and root dimensions are larger and are wider until the incisal edge, and its asymmetric characteristics, which helps differentiate between its counterpart and the location of the hemi-arch to which it belongs (TEXEIRA).
It has a length of 22.0 mm and an ascending series in the lower incisors and a descending series in the upper incisors (TEXEIRA, 2001).
The arrangement of teeth as well as the occlusion scheme is divergent among individuals (KUMARI, FIDA and SHAIKH, 2016). Normally, the Lower Lateral Incisor (ILI) is located parallel between the distal face of the lower central incisor and the mesial face of the lower canine. Being the second tooth of each hemi-arch with similar characteristics to the lower central incisor, however the ILI (32 and 42) show increased size in all dimensions (TEXEIRA, 2001) (Fig. **X**).

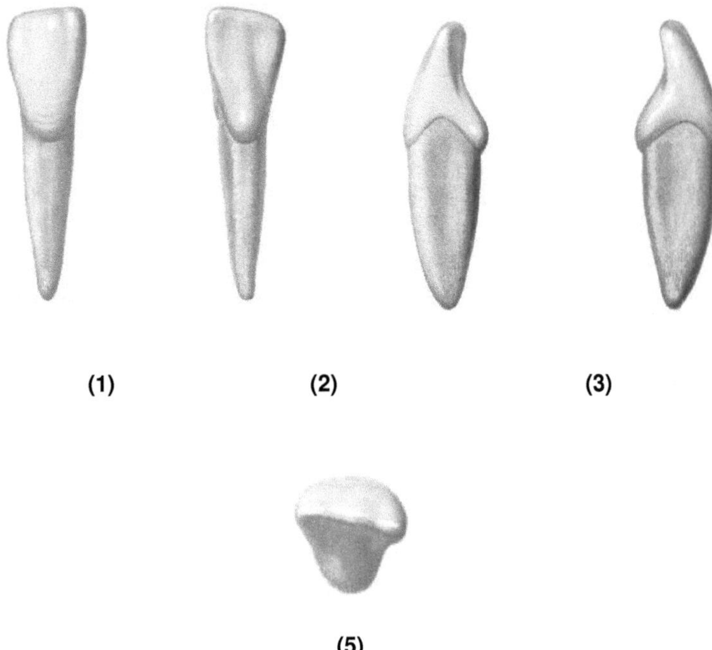

(1)   (2)   (3)

(5)

Figure X - Anatomy of the permanent right mandibular lateral incisor (42). **1** - Buccal face; **2** - Lingual face; **3** - Mesial face; **4** - Distal face; **5** - Incisal edge.

CROWN

VESTIBULAR SIDE

The buccal surface is similar to the buccal surface of the mandibular central incisor, differing for being asymmetrical and larger, with mesial and distal edges converging towards the cervical, showing a triangular aspect. It is almost flat in the incisal thirds and convex in the cervical third. The disto-incisal angle is more rounded, unlike the mesio-incisal angle, which is higher and more acute (TEXEIRA, 2001; MADEIRA, 2004).

LINGUAL FACE

The lingual surface has similar aspects to the vestibular surface, being smaller, with anatomical accidents not very evident. The marginal ridges are not voluminous and the cingulum is poorly visualized, there is no blind foramen and the fossa is not evident (MADEIRA, 2004).

PROXIMAL FACES

The proximal faces of the ILI are more convex and with greater inclination, resembling the central incisors, however smaller. Displaying a triangular shape, with a narrower base. The mesial proximal surface is longer and flatter than the distal proximal surface, thus almost parallel, presenting almost rectilinear mesial and distal angles. They are symmetrical with convergence of the distal angle to cervical (OGAWA, C. M. *et al.*, 2016; MADEIRA, 2004).

INCISAL BORDER

The incisal edge of the ILI is wider than the lower central incisor, showing greater inclination to the mesial edge, arising from the mesio-distal inclination, due to the difference in height of the proximal mesial and distal faces. In young people it is noted the presence of three protrusions, popularly known as mamelons that will be worn naturally (MADEIRA, 2004).

COLO

It has the same anatomical aspects of the lower central incisor (TEXEIRA, 2001).

ROOT

The inferior lateral incisor is unirooted. Compared to the root of the central, it is larger in all dimensions, being longer, more robust and presenting deeper grooves, especially the distal one (MADEIRA, 2004). The root is usually deviated to the distal, highlighting a reentrant angle between the distal faces of the crown and root (TEXEIRA, 2001).

ERUPTION

The eruption occurs around 7 years of age, the beginning of calcification is 3 to 4 months, complete amelogenesis between 4 to 5 years and complete rhizogenesis between 10 to 11 years. Its occlusion is with the distal third of the central incisor and the mesial half of the upper lateral incisor (TEXEIRA, 2001).

REFERENCES

MADEIRA, M. C. Anatomia do Dente. 3. ed. São Paulo: Sarvier. 2004. TEIXEIRA, L. M. S.; REHER, P.; REHER, V. G. S. Anatomia Aplicada a

Odontologia. Rio de Janeiro: Guanabara Koogan, 2001.

OGAWA, C. M. *et al.* Mesiodistal width and proximal enamel thickness of lower incisors. **Orthodontics**. v. 49, n. 2, p. 151-159, 2016.

KUMARI, N.; FIDA, M.; SHAIKH, A. Exploration of variations in positions of upper and Lower incisors, overjet, overbite, and irregularity Index in orthodontic patients with dissimilar depths of Curve of spee. **Journal of Ayub Medical College**. v. 28, n. 4, p. 766-772, 2016.

SAM. Atlas of Dental Anatomy, 2020.

CHAPTER 2 - MORPHOLOGICAL CHARACTERISTICS OF PERMANENT CANINES

Valéria Larissa Costa Oliveira Beatriz Simone Monteiro de Melo Daniela Vasconcelos Silva
Maria Luysa Almeida da Silva Allane Rafaella da Silva Quirino
Yasmim Christynne Oliveira Reis de Freitas

Matheus Andrade Rodrigues Gustavo Correia Basto da Silva

GENERAL CHARACTERISTICS

The canine group is located in the anterior portion of the dental arches, after the incisors. It is composed of four teeth, two maxillary (upper) and two mandibular (lower). Together with the incisors form the group of anterior or labial teeth. Its nomenclature is according to the arch it belongs to (upper or lower) and the side of the arch where it is located (right or left).

The canines are teeth with a pointed shape, considered the longest of all teeth. In addition, they have a more yellowish color than the others because they have a greater amount of dentin in their composition.

CANINE FUNCTIONS

The main function of the canines is to tear the most resistant foods, mainly due to their pointed morphology that resembles a spear. In addition to this function, they are also important for grasping food and objects in the mouth; for maintaining the lip position, essential

for aesthetics; and for a good fixation in oral rehabilitations (implantodontics, orthodontics, among others), due to their long and resistant roots.

MORPHOLOGY

Crown

It presents five faces: vestibular, lingual, occlusal, distal and mesial. It has the shape similar to the tip of a spear, because in its occlusal edge displays an angulation, characterizing a pointed cusp, which has an important role in the laceration of food. (TEXEIRA, 2008).

Root

The canine group are in general unirradiculated, presenting the conic-pyramidal format, being a long and resistant root (TEIXEIRA, 2008).

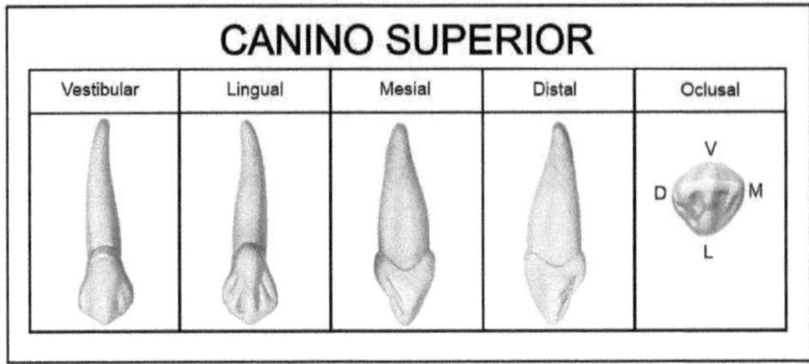

Fig. 2.1. Right upper canine GENERAL

The upper canine is situated just after the lateral incisor in each upper hemi arch. It is considered the most resistant and the longest of all teeth, with a total length of approximately 26.5 mm. Its eruption happens around 11 years of age. The upper canine will establish an occlusion with half of the distal face of the lower canine and half of the mesial face of the lower first premolar.

CHRONOLOGY AND DIMENSIONS OF THE UPPER CANINE

The calcification period begins around the fourth to fifth month of life, by six to seven years of age, the process of amelogenesis is already complete, its eruption occurs between eleven and twelve years of age, and from thirteen to fifteen years of age the rhizogenesis is already complete (TEXEIRA, 2008).

The maxillary canine has a total length of 26.5 mm, with possible variations in size ranging from 20.0 to 35.5 mm. The length of the crown can also vary, ranging from 8.2 to 13.6 mm, and its root varies from 10.8 to 25.1 mm.

CROWN

VESTIBULAR SIDE

The buccal aspect of the crown of tooth 13 or 23 has a cusp on the incisal and pentagonal shape. The cusp has a smaller mesial edge and a longer distal edge inclined towards the cervical. The bridge of this cusp is centered on the imaginary long axis of the tooth (MADEIRA, 2010). The mesial and distal edges of the cuspid are at an almost right angle, more specifically at an angle
of approximately 105º. The mesial side of the crown is convex in the middle third and becomes flattened near the cervical line. The distal side of the crown in the vestibular view is "S" shaped or sinuous or also called sigmoid (TEIXEIRA, 2008). The labial ridge, elevation of the buccal surface, also called buccal ridge, is prominent in the middle and incisal thirds. Bordering laterally this ridge, there are two development depressions that are shallow, one in the

mesial and another on the distal. The contact areas on the mesial side are at the junction of the incisal and middle thirds and on the distal side a little more displaced towards the cervical side, closer to the root than to the mesial side of the crown. The apical third is narrower from mesial to distal, so the root is wider at the cervical side and tapers toward the root apex, while the apical third is narrower from mesial to distal. The apex of these teeth is rounded or may be slightly acute, another possibility is the apical third of the root is slightly tilted distally (TEIXEIRA, 2008; MADEIRA, 2010).

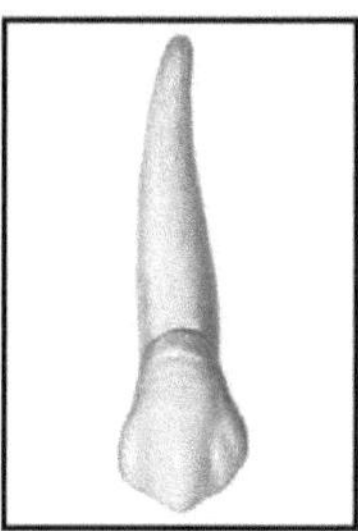

LINGUAL FACE

The lingual surface of maxillary canines is smaller than the buccal surface. It has a large and centralized cuspid, a key feature to differentiate upper from lower canines (MADEIRA, 2010). The tip of the cuspid is centered on the imaginary long axis of the tooth. There is also a lingual ridge that is centralized and prominent, joining the incisal edge and the
cingulum. Furthermore, there are two marginal ridges, a longer and straight one which is the mesial and a shorter, curved and elevated one which is the distal. The presence of shallow fossae in the mesial and distal lingual ridges can be noted. The root seen from the lingual aspect, is this narrower than the buccal (TEIXEIRA, 2008; MADEIRA, 2010).

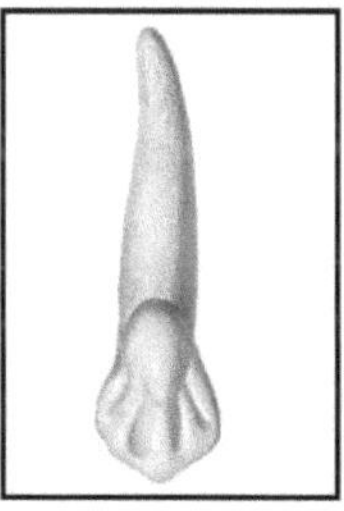

MESIAL FACE

The mesial proximal face is wedge-shaped or "V" that favors the penetration of the crown of these teeth in food which will facilitate its main function which is cutting and drilling these foods (MADEIRA, 2010). The tip of the cuspid is bulky, this tip of cuspid, formed by the junction of the buccal and lingual ridges, is quite resistant since the large amount of enamel.

As in the other maxillary anterior teeth, in the mesial view of the canines, the incisal edge projects to the buccal aspect in relation to the imaginary axis of the tooth in the proximal view (TEIXEIRA, 2008). The buccal surface of maxillary canines seen from this aspect is more curved than the incisors. The greatest curvature of the cervical line or amelocementary line occurs in the mesial surface, which invades more the crown than the distal surface of upper canines. The root has a large bucco-lingual dimension, especially in the cervical third of the root and smaller in the middle third and apical region. Moreover, it is broad and vertically depressed. The buccal root contour is less convex than the lingual contour (TEIXEIRA, 2008; MADEIRA, 2010).

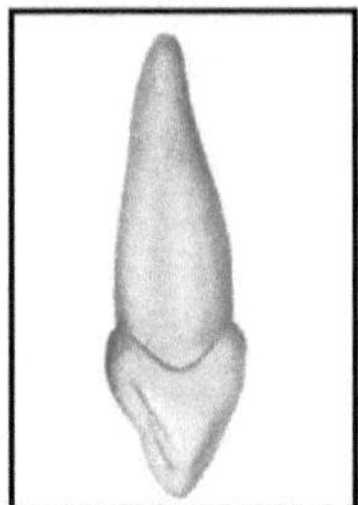

FACE DISTAL

Same crown as the distal aspect, but with less curvature of the cervical line. Furthermore, it is convex cervical to the contact area. On this side, the root has evident width in the cervical and middle thirds. There is also a more pronounced longitudinal depression (MADEIRA, 2010).

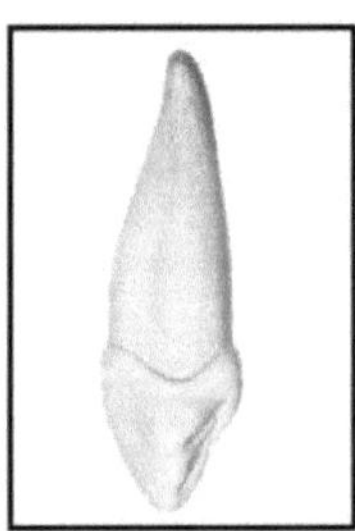

OCLUSAL FACE

This is angled and a greater mesio-distal dimension can be observed for the distal. The largest dimension is vestibulo-lingual on the mesial. In general, the crown on this side has greater bucco-lingual dimension than mesio-distal. It has two slopes, mesial slope: more straight and more horizontal and distal slope: more rounded oblique and larger. It presents bulky and centralized cingulum and its surface is convex towards the vestibular. The lingual ridge divides the lingual face in half, with a shallow pit on each side (TEIXEIRA, 2008; MADEIRA, 2010).

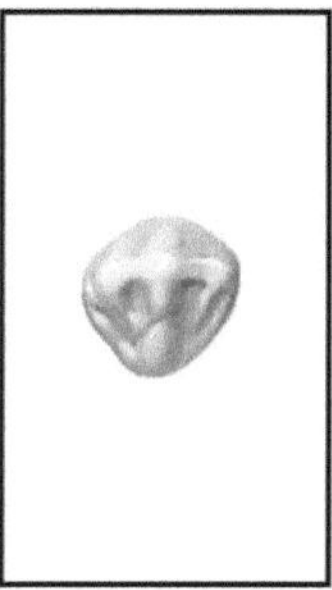

COLO

The neck has a sinuous line and the buccal and palatal surfaces have a semi-circle (MADEIRA, 2010).

ROOT

It has no bifurcation, is straight, conical and pyramidal with angulation towards the vestibular and distal, and also has an inclination towards the distal (MADEIRA, 2010).

Fig. 2.1. Right upper canine

CANINO INFERIOR

Vestibular	Lingual	Mesial	Distal	Oclusal
				V D M L

Fig. 2.2. Right mandibular canine

GENERALITIES

The lower canine when compared to the upper canine is smaller in all dimensions. It is located between the lateral incisor and the first premolar and is the third tooth in the lower hemi arches. It makes occlusion with the distal half of the lateral incisor and the mesial part of the upper canine. In addition, they have a narrower crown, a mesio-distal flattening and a thinner root (TEIXEIRA, 2008; MADEIRA, 2010).

The total length is approximately 25.5 mm. Regarding its eruption, this process tends to happen around 9 years of age.

CHRONOLOGY

As cited by Teixeira, the onset of calcification occurs around 4 to

5 months, the process of tooth enamel formation (amelogenesis) is completed around 6 to 7 years of age, usually the tooth erupts into the dental arch at 9 years of age and the process of root formation (rhizogenesis) is completed between 12 and 14 years of age.

CROWN

According to Teixeira, the general characteristics of this tooth are similar to those described for the upper canine, with smaller size in all dimensions. It is shaped like a pentagon, the crown is longer and narrower as a result of a mesio-distal flattening, which gives it this appearance. It also has a greater inclination towards the lingual side when compared with the crown of the upper canine. Finally, its crown length is 6.9 mm mid-distal and 7.8 mm bucco-lingual.

OCCLUSAL EDGE

The occlusal edge is angled and forms a cusp. It has a smaller buccal-lingual diameter when compared to the edge of the upper canine, as well as their slopes are more asymmetrical (TEXEIRA, 2008)

The apex present in the cuspid is centered on the root. Furthermore, the wear caused by masticatory forces determines an inclined plane for the buccal surface from
of the cuspid, in the shape of a bevel.

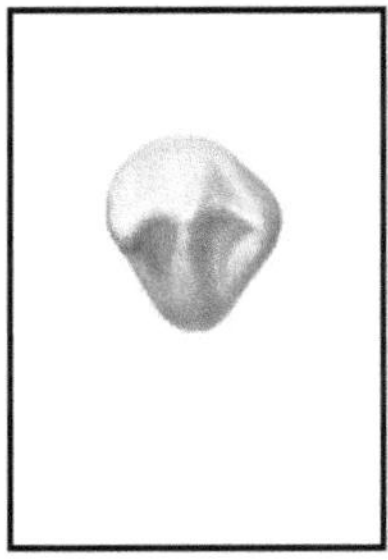

VESTIBULAR SIDE

The buccal surface is convex and has a rectangular shape. This face is higher than the lingual face because the cervical side has a greater descent towards the root than the lingual side. The occlusal edge is formed by two slopes and displays greater asymmetry when compared with the upper canine. The union of these slopes are responsible for forming the angles disto-occlusal and mesio-occlusal (TEIXEIRA, 2008;
WOOD, 2010). On the buccal surface of the upper canine, the mesial side is more rectilinear, with less inclination and longer than the distal side. The distal side has a more convex region, located closer to the occlusal edge, and another more rectilinear and sometimes concave region, found near the cervical bone. Finally, it is on this side that is found, in the cervical third, small longitudinal striations called periquimaceous (MADEIRA, 2010).

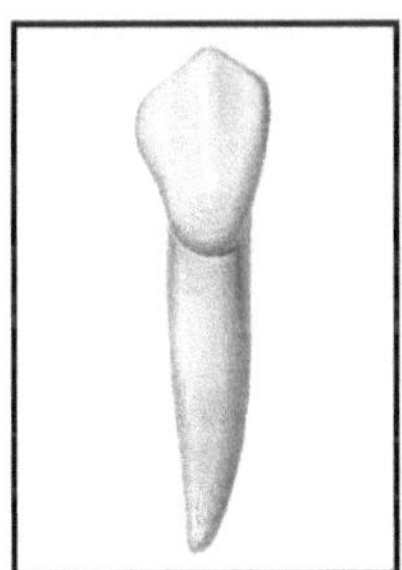

LINGUAL FACE

According to Madeira, in this face the same anatomical elements that are present in the upper canine are also presented in the lower canine, however, less accentuated. With the rectangular shape, the cingulum, the central fossa and its marginal ridges are all little marked and without much definition.

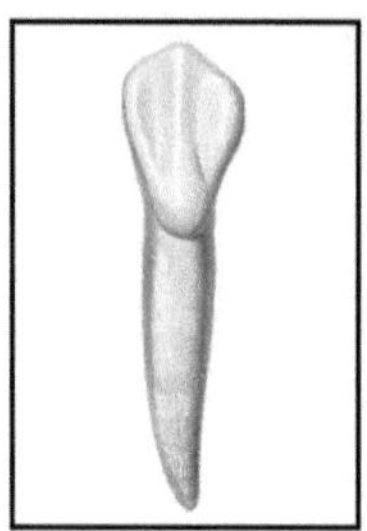

PROXIMAL FACES

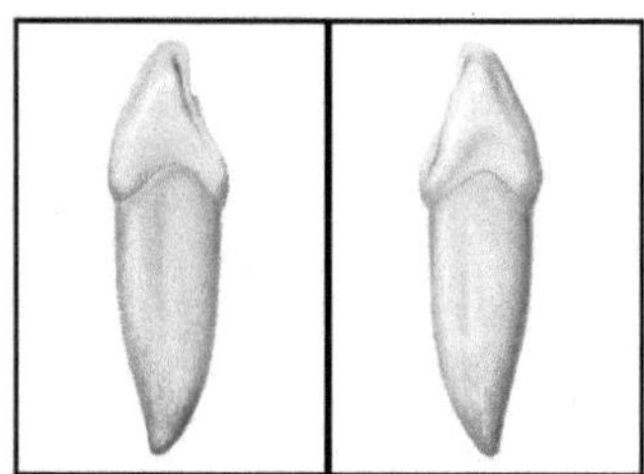

COLO

They have similar format to a triangle, with base located in the cervical region and the apex in the occlusal region. These faces have convergence to the cervical and the mesial face has less convexity and is less inclined compared to the distal face (Wood, When compared to the upper canine, has an oval configuration under the view of a cross-section, and has a depression in the mesio-distal part. Moreover, the anatomical features described are very similar, with smaller curves and more closed angles, except the cervical line, whose position is different in the free faces, since in the buccal face the line is more positioned to apical than the palatal face (TEIXEIRA, 2008)

ROOT

Its root is smaller than the upper canine, has more pronounced mesio-distal flattening and total length of 15 mm (TEIXEIRA, 2008; MADEIRA, 2010).

According to Teixeira, in most cases the root of the lower canine may be single and in some exceptions may contain two roots (about 6% of cases), which concerns a vestibular root and lingual root, being the vestibular root relatively larger, this bifurcation is more frequent in the middle third (MADEIRA, 2010), but can occur in the apex or the entire body of the root (TEIXEIRA, 2008). In relation to the other roots of the lower arch, it is considered the longest and most resistant, in the proximal faces it gives a more robust anatomy with longitudinal grooves. In vestibular and lingual faces the root apex besides being more truncated, it converges to the distal direction. (TEIXEIRA, 2008; WOOD 2010).

REFERENCES

MADEIRA, M.C. **Anatomy of the tooth**. 5ª Ed. São Paulo. Editora Savier, 2010.

TEXEIRA, L.M.S.; REHER, P.; REHER, V.G.S. **Anatomy aplicada à Odontologia**. 2ª Ed. Rio de Janeiro, 2008.

SAM, **Atlas of Dental Anatomy**

CHAPTER 3 - PREMOLARS: CONCEPTS, MORPHOLOGICAL AND FUNCTIONAL ASPECTS

Roger Gabriel Karpowicz Menezes Bruna da Vera Cruz Guedes Camila Moura Maia Dornelas Camila Ketlly Duarte Marinho David Bezerra dos Santos Filho Maria Ismaela Lima de Barros Dias
Patrícia Silva Ferreira Mateus Andrade Rodrigues Gustavo Correia Basto da Silva

The premolar group is exclusive of the permanent dentition, also called the small molar group or bicuspid teeth group, it is formed by the first premolars and upper and lower second premolars; composed of a total of eight teeth - four in each arch; two in each hemiarchus.

FUNCTION

The main function of premolars is to break up and grind food. This is because the first premolars, which are located just after the canines, have an elongation of the buccal cusp similar to the canines, which helps in the tearing function. The second premolar is located closer to the molars, and resembles them, and is suitable to the function of grinding food.

MORPHOLOGY

These teeth are similar to each other, but have unique characteristics. The maxillary first premolars are larger than the maxillary second premolars. The opposite occurs with the mandibular teeth, the first premolars are smaller than the second premolars.

CROWN

The crown of the premolars has a cube shape due to the development of the lingual lobe. Generally they have two cusps: buccal and lingual. The mandibular first premolar can be uni cuspidated, only one root and the second premolar tricuspidated, three roots.

ROOT

All elements of the group are unirradicular except the maxillary first premolar which is usually birradicular. It has a conical pyramidal shape. The roots of the upper ones are flattened in the mesio-distal direction and the lower ones are rounder.

- **UPPER FIRST PREMOLAR (14) (24)**

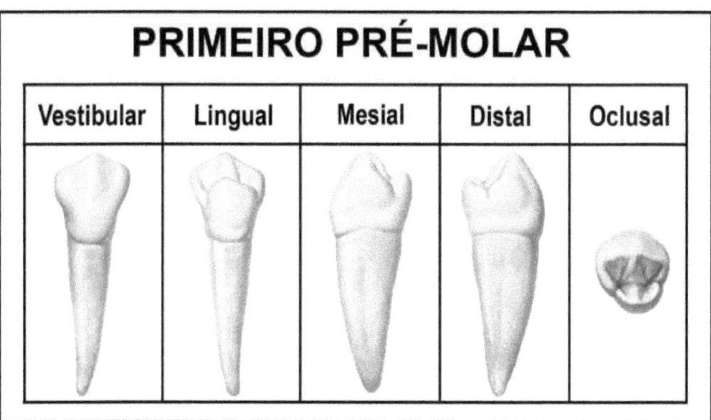

The maxillary first premolar is located just after the canine and is the fourth tooth of one of the upper hemiarcs. Its eruption happens at the beginning of puberty, around 10 years of age.

CROWN

It has the occlusal surface with pentagonal outline (in some cases can resemble a cube), with two cusps, being the vestibular higher and wider than the palatal. Cusps separated by a straight and long groove, with palatal displacement.

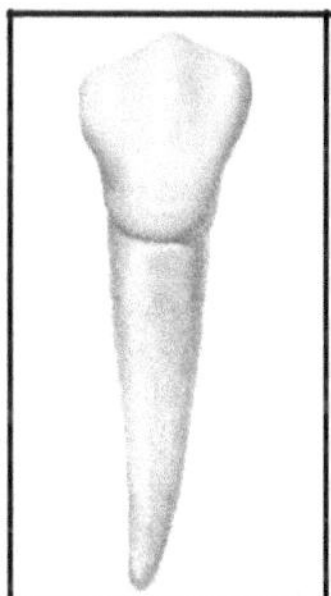

Vestibular face

The buccal surface is similar to the upper canine, although its grooves and convexities are less developed. It is more convex than the canine and also presents a diamond shape, which is wider. The cervical side is rounded with the concavity towards the crown. The proximal sides of the buccal surface are convex and convergent to the cervical. The only great difference in the format, between it and the canine, is in the mesial segment of the longitudinal edge of the cuspid because in the maxillary premolar it is longer than the distal segment of the same cuspid. In the canine, this happens in the opposite way.

Palatal face

Losangular in shape, it has the same contour as the buccal surface, but is smoother, more convex and smaller in all dimensions. Because it is smaller, the contour of the buccal surface can be visualized by the lingual aspect. Since this face is formed by only one lobe, it does not have longitudinal grooves. The occlusal side is formed by two slopes of the lingual cusp. Since they are asymmetrical, the apex of the cusp is displaced from the lingual part to mesial in relation to the midpoint of the crown. completely convex

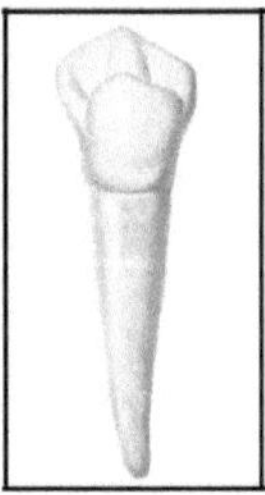

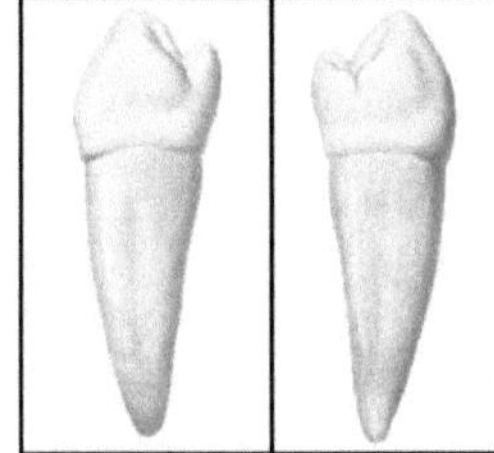

Proximal faces

They have the shape of an asymmetric trapezoid with the largest base located cervically. Their edges (vestibular and lingual) are almost parallel, converging to the occlusal surface. The lingual edge is more inclined and convex. The buccal cusp is the highest and most voluminous. It also has a distal face

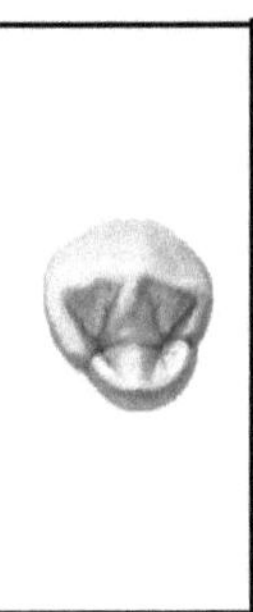

Occlusal face

It is shaped like an asymmetrical pentagon and is less angulated, more oval and with a greater buccal width. For having a lingual face smaller than the buccal, the mesial and distal edges are convergent to it. Its cusps are connected by the mesial and distal marginal ridges, one straight and the other convex, respectively. The groove that separates the cusps is straight and gently displaced towards the lingual side. It has a

fossa called "triangular fossa", because it is formed by the union of three

grooves.

ERUPTION PERIOD

Generally, the maxillary first premolar eruption starts around 10 years of age (beginning of puberty).

ROOT

It usually has two distally inclined, conical-shaped roots. There are cases where these roots are fused, leaving the tooth with an appearance

unirooted. In about 3% of cases, the buccal root is divided in two, giving the tooth a third root.

- **UPPER SECOND PREMOLAR (15) (25)**

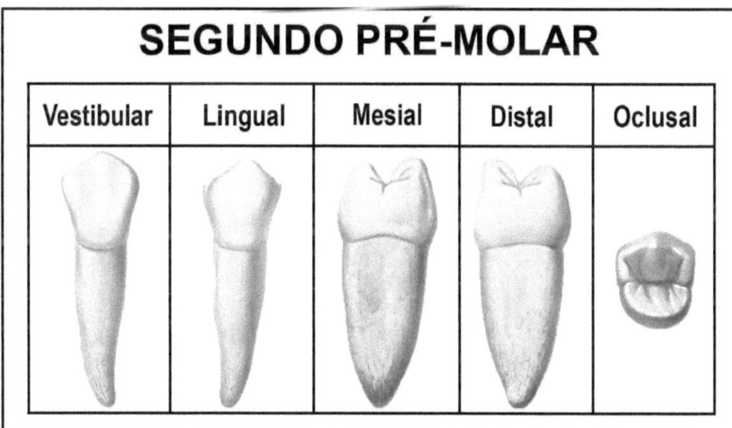

The maxillary second premolar is situated to the distal side of the first premolar, and to the mesial side of the maxillary first molar; in that order, it is the fifth element in the dental arch.

CROWN

It is similar to the first premolar, but is smaller in all directions and has less marked descriptive elements (elevations and depressions). Its more rounded angles give the buccal and lingual surfaces an ovoid rather than angular appearance.

Vestibular face

The buccal surface is morphologically similar to the buccal surface of the maxillary first premolar, but slightly smaller.

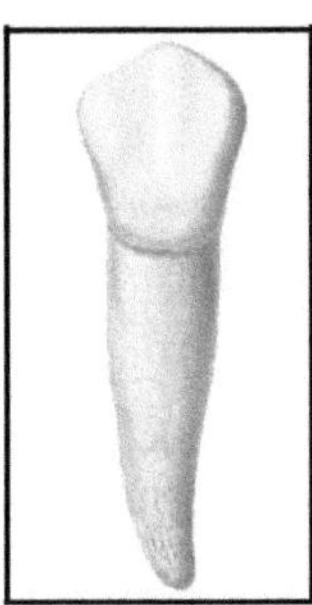

Palatal face

The palatal surface is similar to the buccal surface, but smaller.

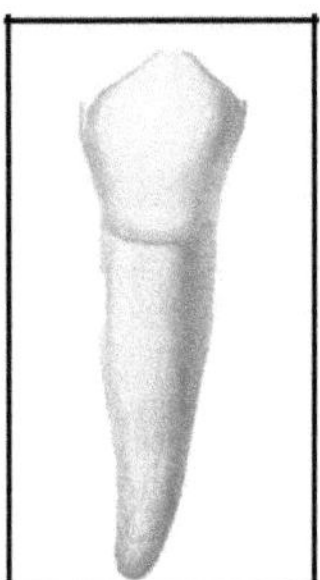

Proximal faces

The proximal surfaces have a quadrilateral shape, with the mesial surface larger and less convex than the distal surface. In the cervical third, these faces are almost flat to maintain the interdental space. In the two occlusal thirds, they are convex to maintain the contact point.

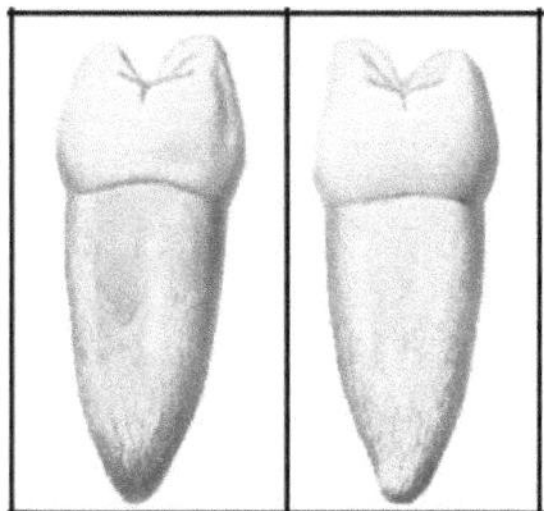

Occlusal face

The contour of the face is oval. The primary sulcus is central and does not move towards the lingual as in the first premolar. The apex of the lingual cusp is aligned with the midpoint of the crown. The difference between the marginal ridges is less accentuated. The mesiodistal diameter on the lingual side is not much larger than on the buccal side.
a striking feature of the maxillary second premolar is the small extension of the main groove in the center of the crown. The mesial and distal fossae will be closer together.

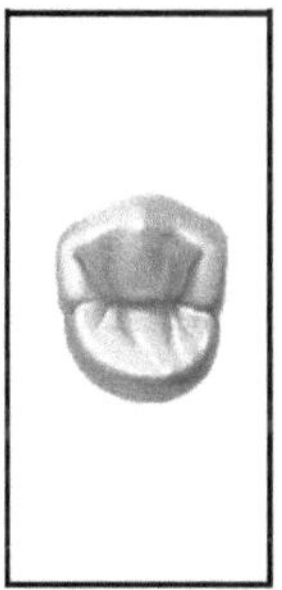

ERUPTION PERIOD

The maxillary second premolar usually erupts between 10 and 12 years of age.

ROOT

The single root, in most cases, is very flattened mesiodistally with deep longitudinal ridges that give its cross-section the shape of a dumbbell.   When not very deep, the section is oval. The length of the roots of both maxillary premolars equals each other.

- **MANDIBULAR FIRST PREMOLAR (34) (44)**

<table>
<tr><th colspan="5">PRIMEIRO PRÉ-MOLAR INFERIOR</th></tr>
<tr><th>Vestibular</th><th>Lingual</th><th>Mesial</th><th>Distal</th><th>Oclusal</th></tr>
</table>

The mandibular first premolar, is the smallest among the premolar group and is located between the mandibular canine and mandibular second premolar teeth. Its occlusal arrangement is formed by the distal of the upper canine and the mesial of the upper first premolar. [2] [3]

CROWN

The crown is cubic-cylindrical in shape and is also bicuspid but its lingual cusp is not very visible.[2]

Vestibular face

The buccal surface is smooth, convex and inclined towards the lingual side. [4] The greatest convexity occurs in the cervical third in the cervical-occlusal direction, forming the buccal boss. The middle and occlusal thirds are strongly inclined towards lingual, decreasing their convexity. In the mesio-distal direction, the middle third has the greatest convexity.[2]

Lingual side

When compared to the buccal surface, it has a smaller size due to the inclination of the lingual surfaces. It has a more regular surface, with a groove coming from the mesial fossa of the occlusal surface, separating the lingual cusp from the mesial marginal ridge. In addition, it has a hump in the mesial-distal direction in the cervical third.[2] [3] [3]

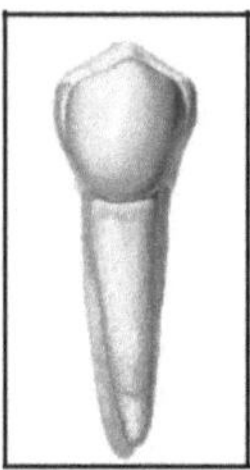

Proximal faces

The proximal surfaces are similar to a trapezoid,[2] their mesial surface is larger and less convex when compared to the distal surface. To maintain an interdental space in the cervical third, these faces are almost flat. And their point of contact is in the convexity located in the two occlusal thirds.[3] The buccal side has a strong convexity, unlike the lingual side where there is less convexity.[2]

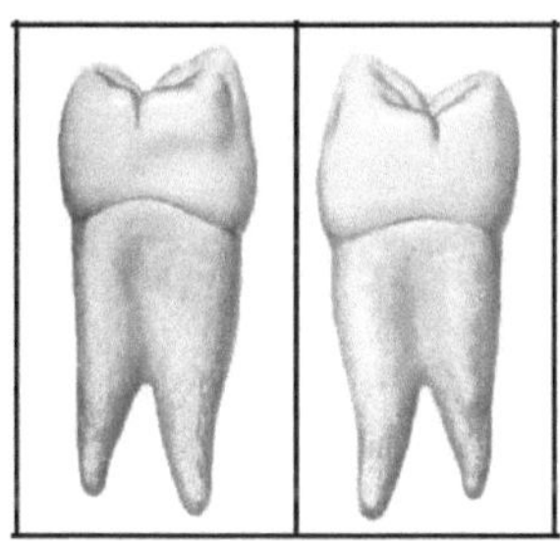

Occlusal face

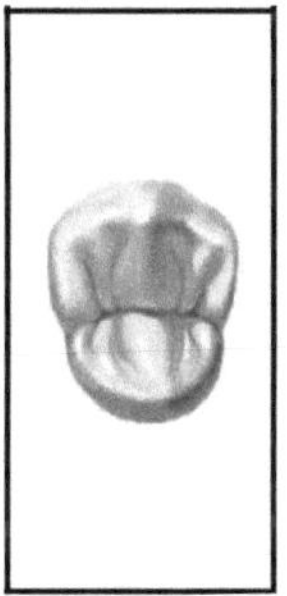

The occlusal surface may vary morphologically, but there are usually standard features found.[2] Thus, this face usually has an oval occlusal with two cusps joined by an enamel bridge, but the buccal cusp is twice as long as its lingual cusp. The main groove is curvilinear and concave towards vestibular.[1] Sometimes, this enamel bridge can be crossed by a central mesiodistal groove in the shape of an arch with buccal concavity.

ERUPTION PERIOD

Generally, the mandibular first premolar erupts completely between the ages of 10 to 12 years. [2]

ROOT

The root of the mandibular first premolar is unirooted and sometimes has a bifurcation at the root apex. In a cross-section, it is flattened mesially and oval or sometimes circular in shape. Moreover, its root inclines distally and can present a complete curvature.[2] Thus, it displays shallow longitudinal grooves on the mesial surface of the root, but rarely deep, cleft-like grooves, which can cause apical bifurcation. [4]

- **MANDIBULAR SECOND PREMOLAR**

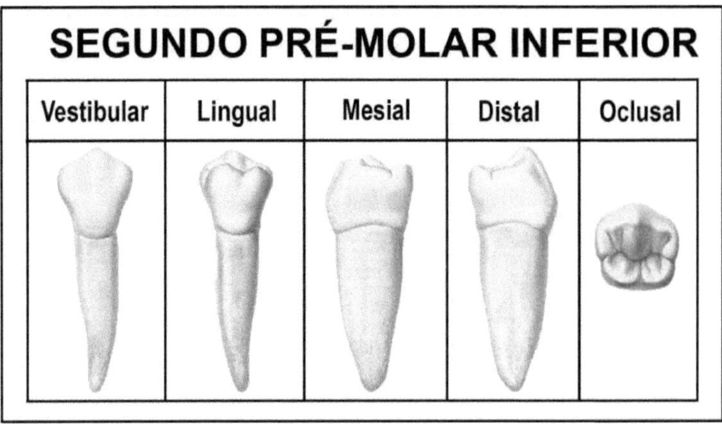

The mandibular second premolar is the fifth tooth of the mandibular hemi-arch and has a more robust anatomy in relation to the mandibular first premolar, with a wider crown and more developed cusps, especially the lingual cusp is located distally to the mandibular first premolar and mesially to the mandibular first molar. In addition, it presents characteristics of transition to molarization that differentiate it from the mandibular first premolar, with more voluptuous aspects and larger dimensions. It is located between the mandibular first premolar and first molar (TEIXEIRA, *et al.,* 2021) and occludes with the distal half of the maxillary first premolar and mesial half of the maxillary first molar (TEIXEIRA, *et al.,* 2021).

Vestibular face

It is more convex, lower and wider than the lower first premolar despite their similarity. It has a more horizontal longitudinal edge and a more rounded cusp. This side inclines towards the lingual side in the occlusal and middle thirds and has a quadrilateral outline because the cusp slopes are not very inclined and the mesial and distal sides are practically parallel. The mesial side is slightly higher, the cervical side has a concavity towards the crown and its occlusal part is the apex of the buccal cusp.

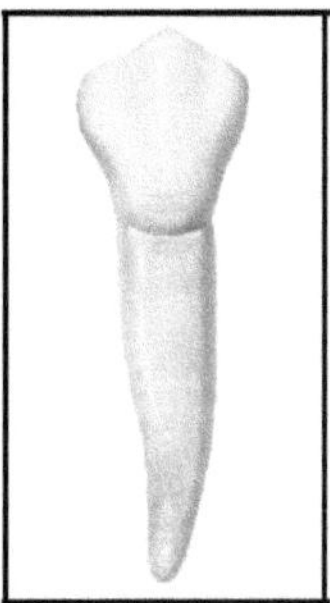

Lingual side

It is possible to see all the cusps of the mandibular second premolar and, when the tooth is tricuspidated, the lingual cusps are divided by a groove originating from the occlusal surface - called the disto-lingual groove because it is located in the distal part of the lingual surface - and separates them into disto-lingual (smaller) and meso-lingual (larger) cusps. It is a surface that is almost as wide as the buccal surface, thanks to its
bulky cusp, but lower than it, besides being convex in all directions. Moreover, it is possible to constantly observe a depression that separates the cusp from the distal marginal ridge.

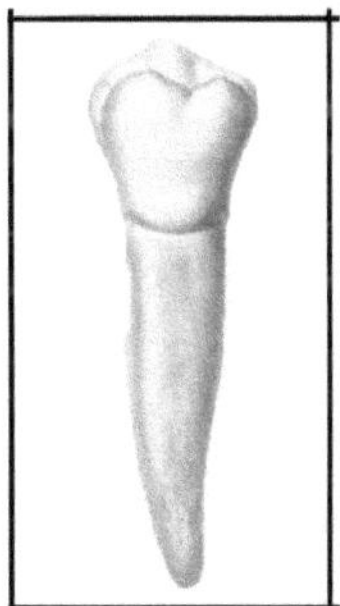

Proximal faces

Divided in mesial and distal, it is possible to observe the difference in size of the lingual cusps, since the faces are proportional to their size. The mesial face is higher and wider than the distal, equivalent to the cusp that outlines it, besides being vaguely less convex. Both are quadrilateral in shape and have the buccal surface inclined towards the lingual surface. The occlusal part houses the masticatory part of the buccal and lingual cusps.

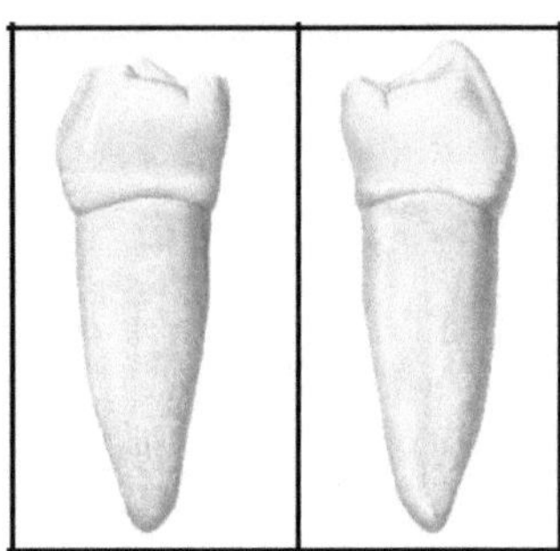

Occlusal face

It has a circular outline, since the buccal and lingual dimensions will be quite similar and bulky, although the mesial and distal marginal ridges converge to the lingual face. It has a variable anatomy, with two more universal forms - the bicuspid and tricuspid.
In the biscuspid format, only one main juice is found, concave in relation to the vestibular, which crosses from the distal side to

The medial juice between the only two cusps - a lingual and a buccal one, which are similar to each other in relation to height, however, the buccal cusp is slightly more voluminous, rounded and has larger dimensions, while the lingual is more pointed. This juice can originate pits that originate secondary grooves in opposite direction to the mesial-distal juice that act limiting the marginal ridges.

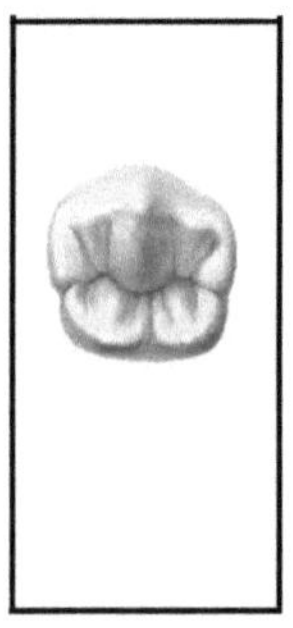

In the tricuspid shape, on the other hand, there is the presence of a deep disto-lingual juice, which originates a bifurcation in the lingual cusp (one mesial and one distal), occurring then the presence of three cusps in the tooth. It presents a main juice of the same shape of the bicuspid plus the disto-lingual juice that derives from it and continues until the lingual face. The union of these juices presents a "y" shape and originates a central fossa.

ERUPTION PERIOD

Generally, the mandibular second premolar has its complete eruption around 11 years of age.
ROOT

It generally has a single, flattened and conical root, which can be circular or oval depending on the cut, with the presence of wide and not very pronounced longitudinal grooves. In buccal view it presents a slight distal deviation and its apex can be rounded or thin and also thick due to the deposit of secondary cementum. In cases of root bifurcation, a buccal and a lingual branch appear with half the height of a single root.

REFERENCES

TEIXEIRA, L. M. S.; REHER, P.; REHER, V. G. S. Anatomia Aplicada a

Odontologia. 2. ed. Rio de Janeiro: Guanabara Koogan, 2001.

MADEIRA, M. C. Anatomia do Dente. 5. ed. São Paulo: Sarvier Editora De Livros Medicos Ltda. 2008.

SILVA, J.A. Guia Curricular para Formação de Técnico em Higiene Dental para Atuar na Rede Básica do SUS. Brasília: Ministry of Health, 1994.

COSTA, A.P.C.; FARIAS, I. A. P.; LEITE, D. F. B. M. Anatomy and Sculpture

Dental. 3. ed. João Pessoa: UFPB, 2020.

SUCIU, Ioana, *et al.* Stereomicroscopic and Microscopic Study of Dental Structural Aspects Derived from Iatrogenic and Pathological Processes Suffered by a Second Mandibular Premolar - A Case Study. **Journal of medicine and life**, Romania, vol. 13, n. 4, p 635-640, Oct./Dec. 2020. Available at: https://pubmed.ncbi.nlm.nih.gov/33456616/. Accessed on: 03 Jan. 2021.

Menegazzo, K., Witti, D., Lazzari, M., Moon, T., Ávila, M., & Dallanora, L. M. (2013). THE **PREMOLAR PREMOLAR PERMANENT GROUP: STRUCTURES ANATOMIC.** *AçãoOdonto, 1*(1),12.Retrieved from https://portalperiodicos.unoesc.edu.br/acaodonto/artcle/view/3783

CHAPTER 4 - ANATOMICAL PROPERTIES OF PERMANENT MOLARS

Lucas Rodrigues dos Santos Amanda Nandyala Menezes Pinheiro Caroline Belisio Leite de Melo
Joycy Pamella Silva Epifanio Kelly Oliveira da Silva
Lucas Vinicius Viana Machado de Santana

Rafaella Soares de Almeida Matheus Andrade Rodrigues Gustavo Correia Basto da Silva

INTRODUCTION

The molars are located in the posterior portion of the dental arch, distally to the premolars. This group is composed of twelve teeth, six in each arch and three in each hemi-arch. The molars are entitled monophyseal teeth because they do not succeed any tooth of the deciduous dentition. They are still considered by some authors as teeth belonging to the deciduous dentition, but with delayed eruption. However, their size and detailed morphology suggest a greater anatomical proximity with permanent teeth than with deciduous teeth. Due to its posterior position in the oral cavity, the molar group can also be called posterior teeth or yaw teeth. They can also be called multi-cuspid teeth or grinding teeth. The molar group is composed of the first, second and third molars. Its nomenclature is based on the position of the tooth in the arch: first molar, second molar or third molar; to which arch the tooth belongs: upper or lower; and to which side of the arch the tooth belongs: right or left. The molars' main function is to grind food. Its multi-cuspidated morphology combined with its posterior position, where muscle strength is more concentrated, allows it to develop an enormous amount of function. Moreover, it is highly relevant as a factor in maintaining the vertical dimension of occlusion. The presence of these teeth prevents the bite closure with consequent protrusion of the mandible, which would lead to premature aging, overloads and occlusal trauma (TEIXEIRA, 2008). The molars present ample morphological detailing marked by the presence of numerous cusps and roots. In both the upper and lower arches, the molars form a descending series, with the first molars larger than the second molars and the second molars larger than the third molars. The molar crowns have a cuboid shape and are usually very bulky. In maxillary molars, the labial-lingual diameter is greater or equal to the mesial-distal diameter. Their occlusal surfaces are formed by four cusps: three larger ones and a smaller one. The largest and most voluminous is the mesio-lingual cusp, which continues through an oblique ridge with the distobuccal cusp. In the inferiors, the mesio-distal diameter predominates over the bucco-lingual. Their occlusal surfaces are formed by four major cusps and generally a fifth minor bucco-distal cusp. With the exception of the third molars, which have enormous morphological variability, all the elements of the molar group are multirooted. The roots are conical-pyramidal, flattened and frequently fused. The maxillary molars have three roots that can measure almost twice the size of the crown: a mesialvestibular root, a distalvestibular root and a palatine root. They are united in a common root implantation base. The mandibular molars have two roots: a mesial root and a distal root. The union of the roots is near the cervical line and the common base is usually short (TEIXEIRA, 2008).

ANATOMICAL DESCRIPTION OF THE MOLARS AND ARCHITECTURAL ELEMENTS OF THE CROWN

With the purpose of describing a specific portion of the tooth, or to locate in it some anatomical detail or alteration
pathological, the tooth can be divided into thirds by imaginary lines. When the lines are horizontal, the crown thirds are: cervical, middle and occlusal. When the lines are vertical, the crown thirds are mesial, middle and distal (dividing the free surfaces) or buccal, middle and lingual (dividing the proximal surfaces). The root is also divided into cervical, middle and apical thirds. In molars, the cervical third corresponds to the radicular bulb (MADEIRA, 2007)

Cuspid is a quadrangular pyramid-shaped protrusion. Of its slopes or inclined planes, two are on the free faces, smooth slopes, and two on the occlusal face, grinding or occlusal slopes. The smooth slopes are separated from the grinding slopes by longitudinal edges. The mesial smooth and triturating slopes are separated from the distal homonyms on the same cusp by transverse edges. The slopes and edges meet at the apex of the cusp. The **marginal ridge** is a blunt linear eminence located on the mesial and distal edges of the occlusal surface of the molars (it extends from the buccal to the lingual cusps). It prevents food particles that must be crushed from escaping from the masticatory area and also protects the contact area by preventing food impaction thereon. The **enamel bridge** is a linear eminence that joins cusps, interrupting a main groove. The best example is that of the maxillary first molar. The **tubercle** is a protrusion smaller than the cuspid, with no defined shape Carabelli's tubercle of the maxillary first molar is constantly found. Small rounded tubercles occur with some frequency on the occlusal surface of third molars and occasionally on other teeth with imprecise locations. The **hump** is a rounded elevation situated between the cervical and middle thirds of the lingual aspect of the molars. The **main sulcus** is an acute, narrow, linear depression that separates the cusps from each other. In its path, there may be developmental defects (incomplete fusion of lobes) that cause lack of enamel coalescence, translated by fissures. It is a site of easy development of caries due to the high susceptibility of residue accumulation and bacteria proliferation. The **secondary sulcus** is a small and shallow depression distributed irregularly and in variable number on the occlusal surfaces, mainly on the cusps and delimiting the marginal ridges. It makes the masticatory surface less smooth, increasing the efficiency of trituration, and serves as an outlet for triturated food. The **main fossae** are depressions found at the termination of the main groove (near the marginal ridges or on the buccal surface) or at the intersection of two of them. In the meeting of a main groove with one or two secondary grooves, secondary fossae (smaller and less deep) are formed. At the bottom of the main fossae small irregular depressions or deep spots in the enamel may appear, known as **scars**. Like fissures, these are elective sites for caries.

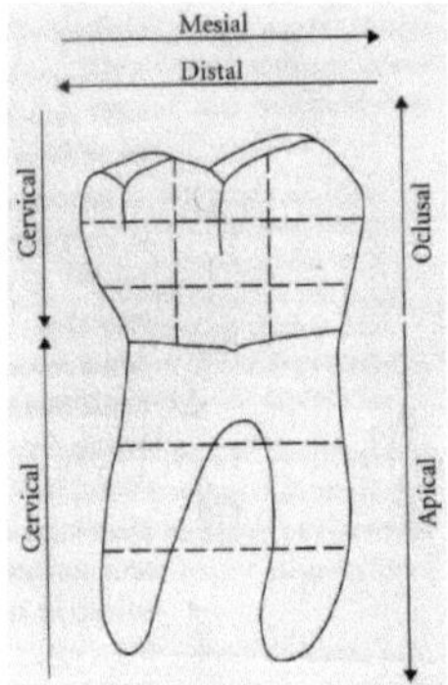

UPPER FIRST MOLAR

The maxillary first molar comprises the elements 16 and 26 in the upper dental arch and has a total length of approximately 20.0 mm. Its eruption usually starts the mixed dentition, which is defined as an intermediate phase between the transition from deciduous to permanent teeth (TEIXEIRA, 2008).

It is located distally to the second upper premolar in the permanent dentition. And, distally to the second deciduous molar, in the mixed dentition. In both dentitions the maxillary first molar corresponds to the sixth tooth in the upper hemiarchus. Its calcification begins around the first month of age and its eruption is around 6 years of age. The upper first molar occludes mesially with the lower first molar and distally with the lower second molar (TEIXEIRA, 2008).

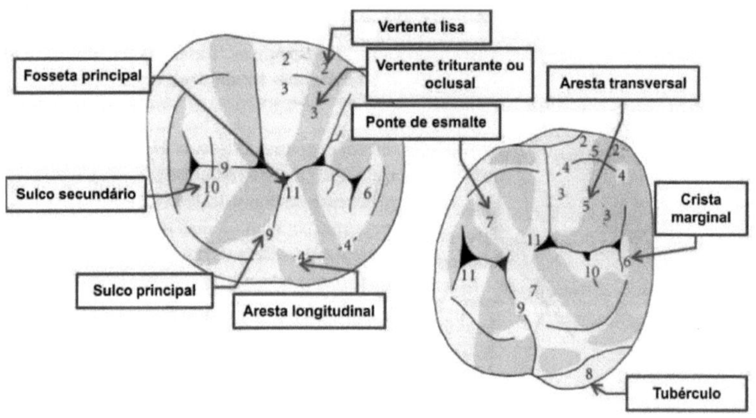

CROWN

The maxillary first molar is composed of buccal, lingual, mesial, distal, occlusal and cervical surfaces. The crown is wide near the junction of the middle and occlusal thirds and narrower near the cervical line.

Vestibular side: It has a trapezoidal silhouette, can be divided into the cervical and mesial occlusal thirds and is convex in all directions. The cervical side corresponds to the smaller base and the occlusal side to the larger base. The cervical border is composed of two curved segments with concavity directed towards the root, separated by an enamel tip. The two proximal edges are highly convergent to the root, the distal edge being smaller and steeper and the mesial edge flatter. The occlusal edge is formed by two segments that converge and have open branches whose apices
correspond to the tips of the buccal cusps. The mesiobuccal cusp is slightly wider and higher than the distal buccal cusp. This face is divided by a buccal groove in two different segments, one mesial and one distal.

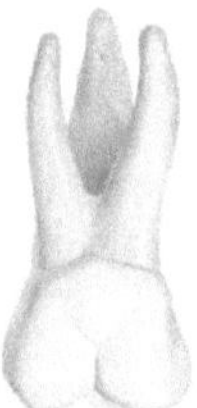

Lingual side: Silhouette similar to the vestibular side, however it has a shorter cervical side and a longer occlusal side. Its cervical edge has a slight curve towards the occlusal side. The proximal edges are similar to the edges of the buccal surface. The occlusal edge is characterized by two segments of different sizes, the mesial one being larger as it corresponds to the mesio-lingual cusp. The surface of the lingual surface is cut by a lingo-occlusal-distal groove that begins in the center of the lingual surface and forms an arch towards the occlusal surface. This sulcus may end in a lingual fossa or may continue straight until it joins the lingual sulcus of the lingual root. This face may present a small tuberosity called "tubercle/Cuspid of Carabelli", in the mesial third.

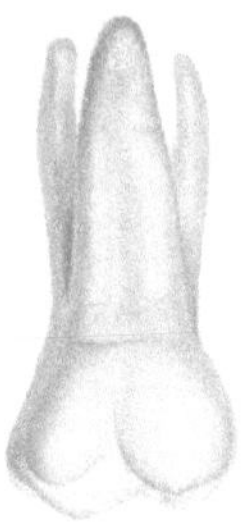

Proximal Faces: These are the widest faces of the crown. Both the mesial and distal faces are rectangular in shape. They show greater convexity near the occlusal surface and may be slightly concave in the cervical third. The buccal and lingual edges are convex, the cervical edge is concave to the root and the occlusal edge has an inverted "V" shape (TEIXEIRA, 2008).

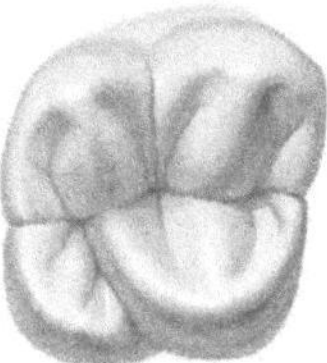

Occlusal Face:

It is characterized by a rhomboidal shape with acute angles in vestibular-mesial and distal-lingual and obtuse angles in distal-vestibular and mesial-lingual. Both the buccal and lingual sides are convex and divided in two rows forming two buccal and two lingual cusps respectively. The proximal sides are convex and converge in the lingual-distal direction.

The cusps have different volumes, the largest volume is the mesio-lingual, followed by the mesiovestibular, disto-vestibular and disto-lingual cusps. The mesi-lingual and distobuccal cusps are joined together by their ridges, forming an enamel bridge (oblique ridge).

The buccal cusps are separated by the vestibulo-occlusion-mesial sulcus, which starts from a central triangular fossa and moves towards the vestibular surface, ending in a small fossa located in the middle third of this surface. While the cusps

The lingual groove is divided by the lingual-occlusion-distal groove, which begins in the distal triangular fossa and is directed obliquely to the lingual face. There is also a transversal sulcus that follows the direction of the major axis of the tooth and unites the central fossa to the lingual-occlusal-distal sulcus. This groove system draws in the occlusal face the shape of the letter *H.*

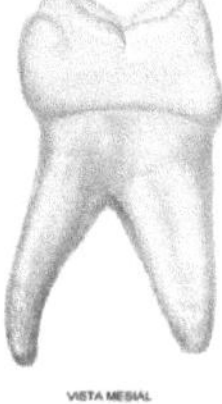
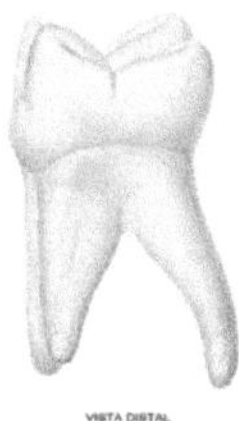

COLO

On the buccal surface, the neck is divided into two portions of concavities facing the root. On the lingual side the neck is convex towards the root and on the proximal side, concave.

ROOT

The maxillary first molar has three roots (tri-rooted) in most cases. The mesial vestibular and distobuccal roots are arranged on the buccal side. And there is the lingual root which is the largest and strongest of the three. They are rarely fused, and if they are, the fusion will happen between the distobuccal and lingual roots, through a cementum bridge.

UPPER SECOND MOLAR
Located between the maxillary first and third molars, the maxillary second molar becomes the seventh element of the hemi-arch. It has a very similar structure to the first molar, but has its own characteristics. Its eruption normally occurs at 12 years of age. Its occlusion is made with the distal third of its lower homonym and the mesial third of the upper third molar.

CROWN

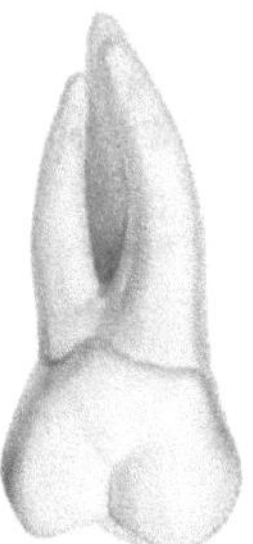

Vestibular side: On this side we notice significant differences from the other teeth, in particular the maxillary first molar, by means of its cusps, such as the mesialvestibular cusp is much larger and more voluminous than the distalvestibular. This great difference in size causes the occlusal edge to be more inclined cervically from mesial to distal. The sulcus that separates the buccal cusps is also smaller and rarely ends in fossettes as in the first molar

Lingual: The upper second molar can be tetracuspid or tricuspid because the distal lingual cusp is smaller compared to the first molar which sometimes disappears. There is neither Carabelli's process nor ridges (in case of absence of distal lingual cusp).

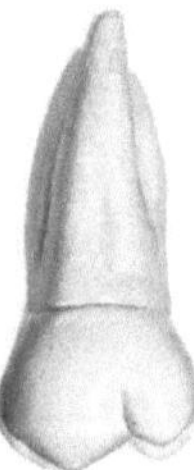

Proximal Face: In cases where the upper second molar is tetracuspidated, the proximal faces are very similar to those of the upper first molar, but with the absence of Carabelli's process. However, when tricuspidated, due to the displacement of the mesial-lingual cusp, the mesial surface is more convex towards the lingual direction and the distal surface is more convex towards the lingual direction, with little distinction between lingual and proximal surfaces.

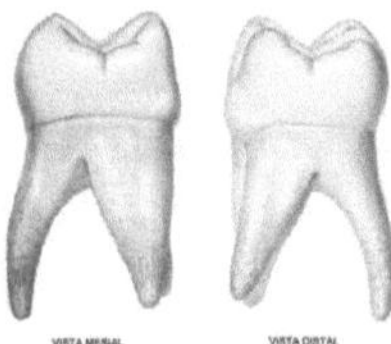

Occlusal surface: Due to the subjectivity of the presence of the disto-lingual cusp, the occlusal surface can have three types: rhomboid, triangular or compression. The rhomboid form, also called rhomboidal, is the most similar to the maxillary first molar, with well-defined cusps, grooves and marginal ridges. However, the presence of secondary grooves, irregularities on the occlusal surface and the mesio-distal flattening form the differences between the two teeth. The triangular form is so called because of the total absence of the disto-lingual cusp. The groove system on the occlusal surface the letter T. The lingual cusp is much more voluminous and higher than the buccal cusps. Finally, the compression form, the least frequent, appearing in less than 10% of cases, in this type of occlusal face the mesio-lingual and disto-lingual cusps are united forming one, giving a long oval aesthetic.

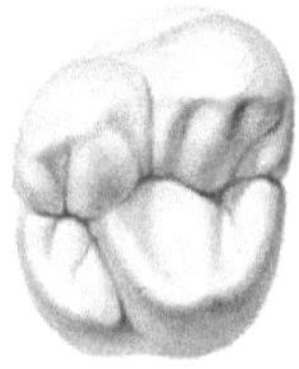

COLO

It has the same characteristics as those presented by the maxillary first molar.

ROOT

The upper second molar is triradiculated, having two buccal roots and one lingual root. The buccal roots are parallel and very close together and incline distally. In 55% the mesial vestibular and lingual roots are distinct, but in 45% they occur to be fused.

UPPER THIRD MOLAR

The upper third molar, more popularly known as "wisdom tooth", is located next to the upper second molar and is the last tooth of the upper dental arch - being understood as element 18 and 28. Its eruption will occur around 18 years of age, being considered the smallest of the upper molars, with a total length of about 17.5 mm (TEIXEIRA, lingual.

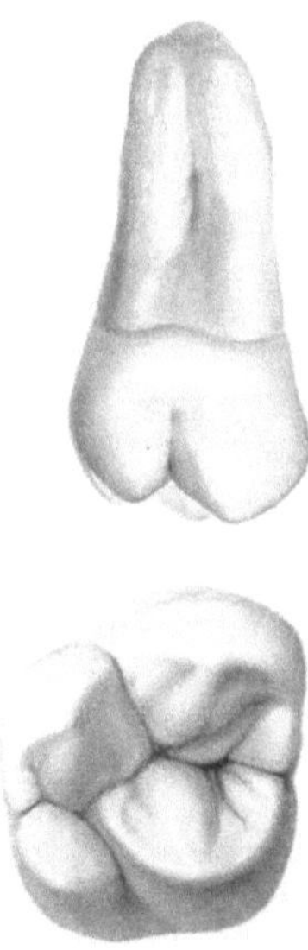

ROOT

Besides, this tooth has a great variability when compared to the other teeth of the hemiarch. Its morphology can go from the simplest to the most complex, not being uncommon to suffer agenesis.

CROWN

The third molar has a standard shape, which is the coronal shape, similar to the tricuspid shape of the upper second molar. Therefore, the differentiation between the third molar and the other upper molars is made by the presence of the numerous grooves on the occlusal surface and the bucco-lingual diameter greater than the mesio-distal. Moreover, Carabelli's tubercle can be foundThe maxillary third molar has three roots, although shorter in length compared to the other maxillary molars, with a more robust inclination and usually fused. In this context, if the 3 roots are fused, the upper third molar will receive the nomenclature of unirradical, having the root a pyramidal shape, with the presence in its lateral faces of longitudinal grooves.
When there is a fusion of two roots, the tooth will be birradicular, in which the fusion usually happens between the lingual and mesial vestibular roots, however, without excluding the vestibular roots and the fusion between the lingual and distobuccal roots, which however rare, can happen. Moreover, the upper third molar can have three roots at the apical level, which in turn is tri-rooted. In some cases, the tooth has four or more roots, therefore being multirooted.

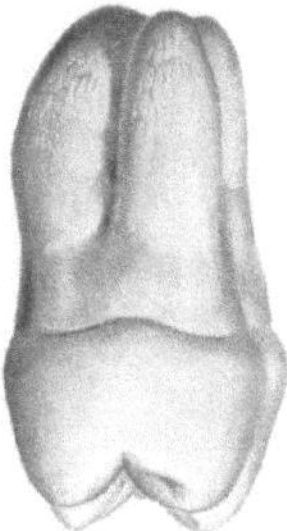

LOWER FIRST MOLAR

The largest tooth in the human mouth with a longitudinal crown, the mandibular first molar erupts in the same age group as the maxillary first molar, at about 6 years of age. In both dentitions (deciduous and permanent), it occupies the sixth position in the hemi-arch, and in the mixed dentition, it is located distally to the deciduous second molar (TEIXEIRA, 2008).

CROWN

About its crown is notoriously robust and shaped like a cube.

Vestibular side: It has a morphology reminiscent of a trapezoid, with the occlusal being the largest base. The cervical is the smallest of the sides and is delimited by the cervical line, this line may present a concavity towards the crown or be more rectilinear. Similar to the upper ones, it may present an enamel tip towards the bifurcation of the roots. As mentioned above, the major base of this "trapezoid" is the occlusal, which is constituted by the vestibular border and the
occlusal, this edge is formed by the 3 most important elements of the vestibular, which are the mesiobuccal, the central vestibular and the distal vestibular cusps. The mesiobuccal cusp is the most robust of all and also the highest, then the mid-vestibular and the smallest of the three is the disto-vestibular. The surface of the vestibular surface is very convex in the cervical third (vestibular hump) and presents a continuation of the mesial and disto vestibular sulci, both sulci are presented cutting the vestibular surface in a vertical way, being the mesial more prolonged, compared to the distal, reaching the middle third of the crown and finishing slightly in the vestibular fossa forming the blind foramen. The disto-vestibular sulcus is smaller and reaches only the occlusal third. It is important to highlight before finalizing that the mesial third can present a tubercle similar to the carabelli, the tubercle of Zuckkandl.

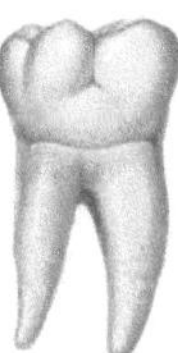

Lingual side: Its contour is similar to the vestibular side, trapezoidal, but is much smaller because the proximal converge to the lingual. The mesial and lingual cusps project towards the occlusal edge (MADEIRA, 2007). Are separated by the lingual buccal groove that is not so imminent, because it has little depth. The mesial side is higher than the distal. The lingual side is more regular, without great variations, besides being convex in all directions.

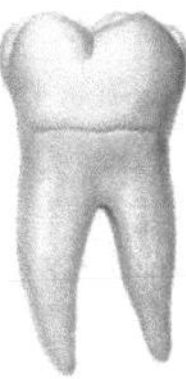

Proximal faces: These are more similar to a rectangle, examining this face it is recognized that there is a lingual inclination of the buccal surface which can be further intensified by the natural physiological wear of age. The cervical side is convex and its concavity is towards the tooth root, as well as the occlusal side which also has concavity that is expressed in the silhouette of the important slopes within mastication as they have a grinding role.

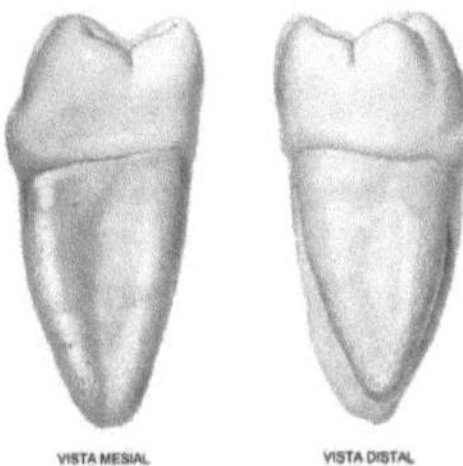

Occlusal surface: It has a morphology that can be compared to a pentagon and is contoured by the buccal, lingual, mesial, distal and vestibular-distal surfaces (TEIXEIRA, 2008). It has greater width in the mesial edge compared to the distal, besides being wider in the buccal edge compared to the buccal edge
lingual. The vestibular face is more elongated, has convexity and includes the grooves and cusps both center-vestibular and mesio-vestibular that intersect this face. In the bucco-distal portion there is the distobuccal cusp, the smallest. The lingual surface is practically parallel to the buccal surface.

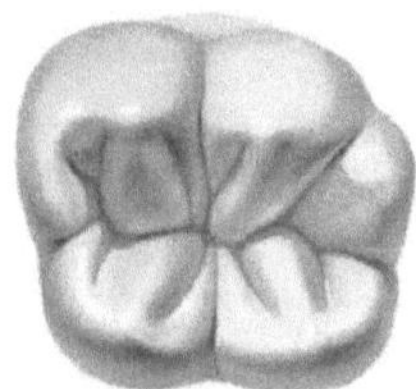

While the proximal edges are more straight and perpendicular. As already mentioned the occlusal surface holds the grooves and cusps, being five cusps in all: two lingual and three vestibular, the cusps plus the mesial of the crown are the largest filling most of it the mesiovestibular for example is the largest of them and soon after the center vestibular. Speaking of the smallest of the cusps we have this vestibular that is present in 95% of the population, if it does not exist the occlusal face is more similar to a rectangle (TEIXEIRA, 2008). The marginal ridges are very clear and will delimit the end of the main medium-distal sulcus. Talking about the grooves, theoretically there are two main ones: buccal-lingual and mesial-distal. The easiest way for these grooves to behave is in a crossed rectilinear manner, but this is not common. Another way that exists is the disposition of the sulcus with three angles that were something similar to the letter "W", it is the most recurrent. The mesial-distal sulcus cuts and divides the buccal and lingual cusps. It begins in the mesial fossa and follows practically straight until the central fossa. From this point on, the sulcus will incline slightly towards the buccal side, separating the central buccal and distal-lingual cusps. From the disto-lingual point there will be a bifurcation of the sulcus, a more robust branch goes towards the vestibular, making the separation between two cusps: disto-vestibular and center-vestibular. The other branch is directed towards the lingual, separating the distobuccal and distal-lingual cusps. The mesio-distal branch reaches even the occlusal vestibular forming the disto-vestibular sulcus.

COLO

As previously mentioned, the neck of this tooth is concave towards the root on the surfaces and/or rectilinear towards the crown on the free surfaces. There may also be indentations both in the cementum toward the crown and in the enamel toward the interradicular sinus.

ROOT

The roots settle based on the crown and form a birradiculated tooth, that is, which has two roots and this occurs in approximately 97.5% of cases (TEIXEIRA, 2008). The two roots that are usually present show parallel to each other, in addition to both have a flattening that moves slightly to mesio-distal and are more widened in the vestibular-distal direction.

LOWER SECOND MOLAR

The mandibular second molar comprises elements 37 and 47 in the lower dental arch and has a total length of approximately 20.0 mm. It is located between the first and third molars, thus becoming the seventh element of the hemi-arch. Its eruption normally occurs at 12 years of age. It occludes mesially with the maxillary first molar, and with the maxillary second molar. Despite the morphological similarity with the lower first molar, they differ because they are a little smaller and have four cusps. The absence of the fifth cusp causes changes in the configuration of the crown (TEIXEIRA, 2008).

CROWN

The mandibular second molar has a crown consisting of 4 cusps and is composed of buccal, lingual, mesial, distal, occlusal and a virtual cervical surfaces.

Vestibular Face: This has a trapezoidal silhouette, with a large occlusal side and convex in all directions. Starting from the cervical third, characterized by the cervical line, which can be rectilinear or manifest a brief concavity. Its buccal groove divides the face into two lobes and ends at the level of the cervical third in a triangular fossula. The mesial lobe is slightly larger than the distal one. This face is smaller than in the first molar due to the presence of only two cusps. In the occlusal edge there is the presence of the projections of the cusps: mesio-vestibular and disto-vestibular (TEIXEIRA, 2008).

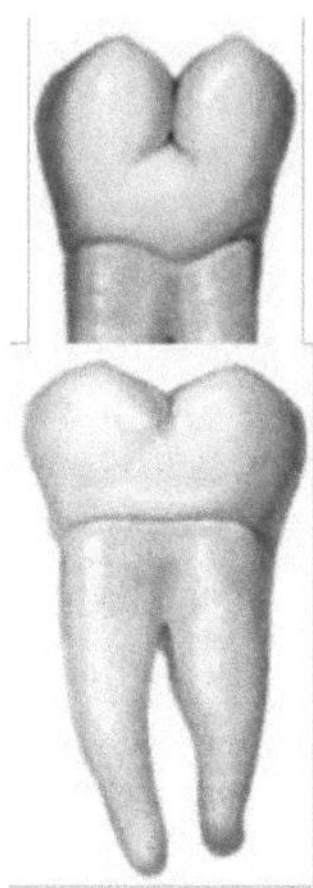

Lingual surface: This has a trapezoidal silhouette and has similar characteristics to the lower first molar. It is more convex and smaller than the buccal surface. Its edges are mesial and distal, mesial is larger and less convergent to the root. The distal edge is smaller and more convergent to the root. The cervical segment has 2 concave segments towards the root, which are joined by a point in the middle third that is inserted between the mesial and distal roots. The occlusal is formed with the apices corresponding to the tips of the buccal cusps. With

Regarding anatomical landmarks, there are no grooves, only a very shallow depression separating the two facial lobes and the lingual boss located in the cervical or middle third.

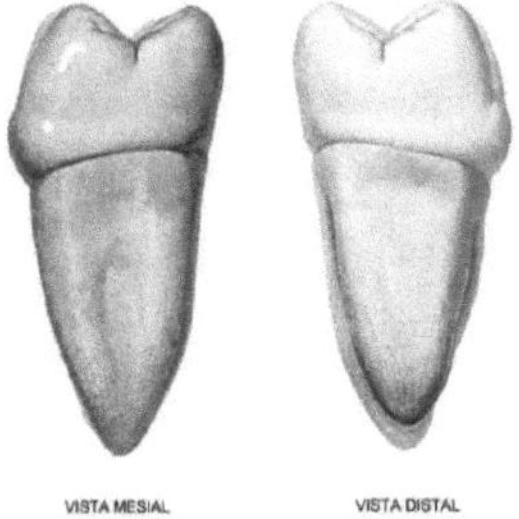

Proximal surface: characterized by a trapezoidal shape, flat on the middle and cervical thirds, the buccal surface diverges toward the root, is rectilinear in the occlusal two thirds, becoming convex in the cervical or middle third, the lingual surface diverges toward the root, is curved, with accentuated L convexity in the cervical or middle third, and the occlusal is V-shaped with a truncated apex by the marginal ridge. The cervical third is characterized by a curvilinear line of concavity towards the root and anatomical landmarks. Its mesial side is larger than the distal side.

Occlusal surface: It is characterized by a rectangular shape, and has four cusps, two vestibular, which are the mesio-vestibular and disto-vestibular, and two lingual, which are the mesio-lingual and disto-lingual. The cusp of larger volume is the mesio-lingual, followed by the mesio-vestibular, disto-vestibular and finally the disto-lingual. There is the presence of two main grooves: the mesial-distal groove and the buccal-lingual groove with a cruciform aspect. Besides the accessory grooves that start from the extremities of the mesial-distal groove towards the mesial and distal faces. In the meeting of the two grooves there will be a central fossa.

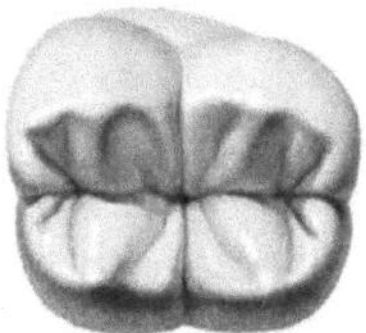

COLO

It presents the same anatomical characteristics described for the first lower molar.

ROOT

The second lower molar is mostly birradiculated, having a mesial root and a distal root, both with the same characteristic of flattening in mesial-distal. They are similar in terms of root characteristics to the lower first molar, but have a greater number of fusion and more adjoined roots (TEIXEIRA, 2008).

THIRD LOWER MOLAR

The lower third molar is located after the second molar, being the last tooth of the lower hemiarchid, understood as element 38 and 48. Its eruption will happen between 16 and 21 years, being the smallest of the lower molars, however more elongated than the upper third molar, with a total length close to 16.00 mm (TEIXEIRA, 2008). As the upper third molar, the lower third molar also presents variations in morphology, but in smaller proportions.

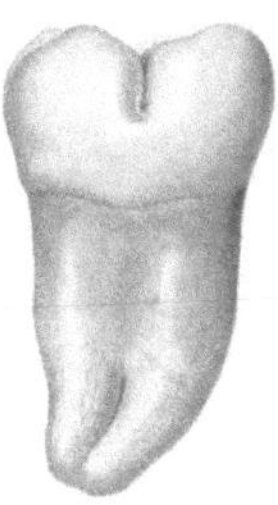

CROWN

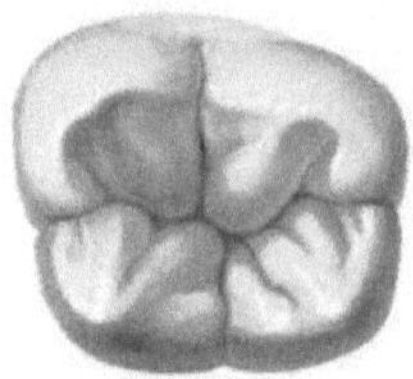

Due to variations in its morphology, the mandibular third molar is described in a manner that differs from the other teeth of the mandibular dental arch. The third molar can be pentacuspidated, which is the most common form of presentation, with a distalized distal cusp, which can replace the distal marginal ridge.
However, less frequently, the mandibular third molar can be tetracuspidated, with the presence of secondary sulci.

ROOT

The roots of the mandibular third molar are disposed to variability, i.e., may present root fusion with distal curvature. In case of total fusion, this root will gain the shape of a quadrangular pyramid. Furthermore, in size, the crown is larger than the root that supports it.

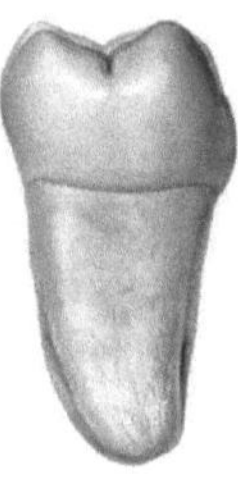

REFERENCES

MADEIRA, Carlos. **Anatomy of the tooth**. 5. Edition. São Paulo. Sarvier, 2007.

TEIXEIRA, L. M. ; REHER, V. G. S. **Anatomia aplicada à odontologia**. 2 Ed. Guanabara Koogan S. A. Rio de Janeiro, 2008.
Sam. **Atlas of dental anatomy**.

CHAPTER 5 - THE USUAL MORPHOLOGICAL STRUCTURE OF DECIDUOUS TEETH

Edlane da Silva Sousa Priscylla Gabrielly Brasileiro de Melo Jhulie Lorrany Mendes de Almeida João Paulo Soares de Oliveira Myllenna dos Santos Ferreira Matheus Andrade Rodrigues Gustavo Correia Basto da Silva

Introduction

Knowledge about the anatomical details and histological characteristics of deciduous teeth is of fundamental importance, either to reestablish shape or function, often resulting from a carious lesion or a

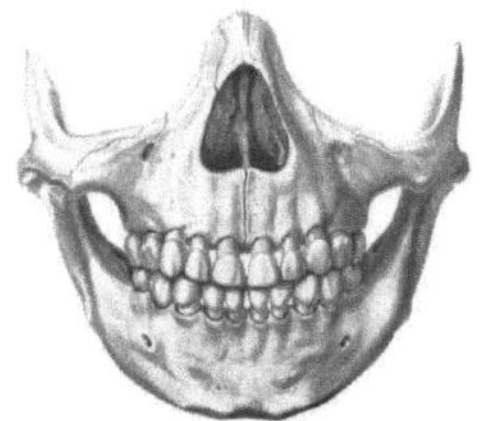

Figure 1 - Anterior view of the child's skull. Relation of the teeth

trauma. Although deciduous teeth present very discrete anatomical characteristics, this group of teeth presents many individual details that will be addressed below.

General

The appearance of deciduous teeth in the oral cavity happens around 6 months of age and total eruption is completed around two and a half years of age. Their replacement by permanent teeth starts to happen after 6 years of age and continues around 11 years of age until the replacement of the last tooth. The deciduous teeth have the same functions as permanent teeth, except for the maintenance of the space necessary for the eruption of permanent teeth. Compared to permanent teeth they are smaller and have a higher degree of attrition. They are arranged in the oral cavity in arches, one upper and one lower, located in the maxilla and mandible through alveoli, and fixed by the periodontal ligament. Among the physiological functions assigned to the deciduous teeth, which are extremely important, we can highlight: mastication, formation of the occlusal plane, maintenance of space, maintenance of vertical dimension, beginning of phonation.

Number of teeth and nomenclature

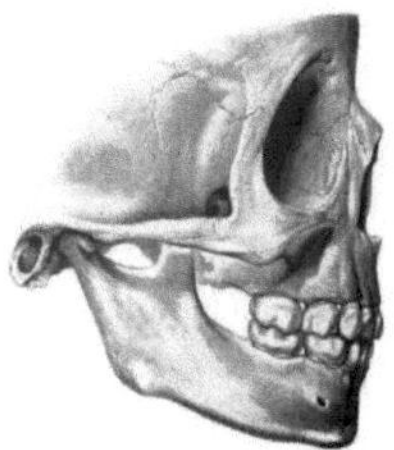

Figure 2 - Lateral view of the skull of a child.

Unlike permanent teeth, deciduous teeth are found in the oral cavity with a total of 20 teeth: 10 in the upper arch and 10 in the lower arch. They are further divided into four hemiarcs, which have 5 teeth each. As far as nomenclature is concerned, there are several known terms, such as: milk teeth, deciduous or first dentition teeth.

Biological Functions

Deciduous teeth have biological functions of mastication, phonetics, swallowing, aesthetics, besides being responsible for maintaining spaces for permanent teeth, containment of antagonists in the occlusal plane and stimulation for maxillary and mandibular development. Knowledge of these details is important and influences both the recognition of deciduous teeth and the dissipation of some difficulties during their rehabilitation. Although deciduous teeth remain in the oral cavity for a short period of time, they are considered excellent natural space conditioners. This helps to avoid problems of reduced arch perimeter, loss of dental space, tooth migration and other factors that contribute to occlusion imbalance. It is therefore important to emphasize that the first molars play an important role during the mixed dentition because it is through them that the first permanent molar is positioned, and it is necessary to maintain these teeth to avoid disharmony in occlusal development.

Early loss of deciduous teeth

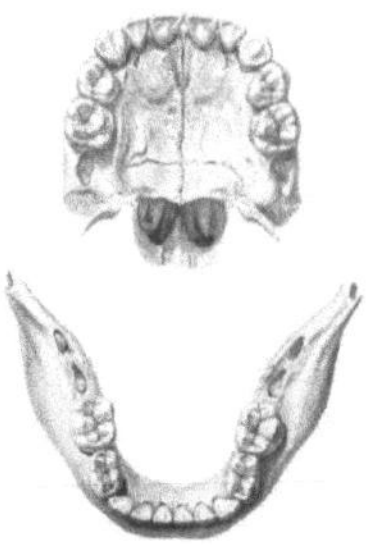

Figure 3 - Occlusal view of upper and lower deciduous teeth.

The loss of a deciduous tooth is considered early or premature when it occurs at least one year before its normal eruption. However, the major causative factor of dental problems in children and adolescents is still the lack of prevention of the dental element and the caries disease not treated correctly. The most common major causes of early deciduous tooth loss are caries, trauma,developmental abnormalities and early root resorption of deciduous teeth. The first years of human beings are important for monitoring oral conditions. It is in this phase of life that one should have the main attention to oral health so that in the future, in adulthood, there is no development of more severe oral problems and the dental element is not removed early. However, if the permanent successor is well developed, after the early loss, its eruption can be accelerated, thus reducing the risk of space loss.

■ Deciduous *versus* permanent Existence of diastemas in the dental arch of the deciduous dentition

In the deciduous dentition, the presence of interdental spaces in the anterior superior regions is normal. The interdental spacing can add up to 10 millimeters with an average of 4 millimeters in the maxilla. Spacing between the deciduous incisors is normal and has been termed physiologic spaces. They are considered desirable for the accommodation of successor teeth, considering that permanent teeth are larger than deciduous teeth. Their presence indicates that the permanent teeth will probably have adequate space when they erupt. Children with archwires with diastemas present a lower tendency of crowding when the permanent incisors erupt. The absence of interdental spaces or the presence of crowding are signs that the permanent incisors probably will not be properly positioned in the arch. In general, deciduous arches with spaces produce a favorable alignment of the permanent incisors.

Teeth size

Deciduous teeth are smaller than permanent teeth. The arch in the permanent ones gives a descending form size (1ºMolar > 2º Molar > 3º Molar), while in the deciduous arch it is ascending (1ºMolar < 2º Molar). The roots of deciduous teeth are smaller, thinner and lighter in color than permanent teeth. The relationship between crown and root in deciduous teeth shows a larger root than crown. In permanent teeth this comparison is not so great. The pulp chamber of deciduous teeth is larger in proportion when compared to permanent teeth and they follow the external morphology.

Color of the teeth

The coloration of the crown of permanent teeth varies from yellowish white to grayish white. The dental enamel is very translucent, revealing the dentine color, which is responsible for the color of the dental crown. Some factors, such as the degree of mineralization, influence the color of teeth, because the more mineralized the teeth are, the darker they will be. We can cite the example of deciduous teeth, whose mineral content is lower and, therefore, are lighter. In the same dental arch, differences in color are observed as the incisors are lighter than the premolars and molars, while the canine, due to its large volume of dentin, appears darker than neighboring teeth. In the same tooth, a darker shade is observed in the cervical third than in the incisal third. With age, teeth tend to become darker due to enamel wear, which makes the dentin more transparent; besides that, chemical and physical extrinsic factors propitiate acquired colorations, such as through smoke and   other and other coloring substances, influencing the teeth color.

■   **Groups of deciduous teeth**

INCISOR GROUP

General

In the human dentition, the incisor group is composed of eight teeth, located in the anterior portion of the arch, two for each hemiarchus. The primary function of this group is chewing, as well as grasping and cutting food. In addition, it plays a relevant role in aesthetics and phonetics.

■   **Superior Central Incisor**

The maxillary central incisor occupies the most mesial part of the upper hemi-arch. It has no mamelons when recently erupted and is the only anterior tooth in which the mesio-distal dimension of the crown is comparatively larger than the cervical-incisal dimension. Thus, its crown is more load than long, but narrow near the neck.

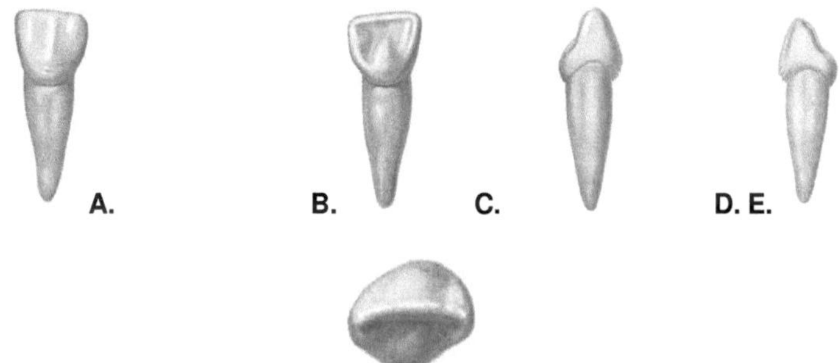

Figure 4 - A. Vestibular face; B. Lingual face; C. Mesial face; D. Distal face; E. Occlusal face.

The incisal edge is very flat and divides the crown into two approximately equal halves: lingual and vestibular. The disto-incisal angle is slightly more rounded and obtuse than the mesio-incisal, which has a more acute angle. The buccal surface is convex and rarely depressed. This side shows a greater mesio-distal dimension than the cervico-incisal side. The incisal side is relatively flat and corresponds to the incisal edge. The cervical side is smaller and convex towards the root.

The mesial and distal sides are more convex than in the central permanent. The mesial side of the crown is very flattened, while the distal side is more convex. The mesial contact area is near the mesioincisal angle; the distal contact area is in the incisal third. On the lingual side the cingulum and the marginal ridges are well accentuated, causing the lingual fossa to be in the incisal third of the lingual side. The proximal surfaces are convex in all directions. The cervical side is pronounced and concave towards the root. The mesial side is similar to the permanent tooth except that it is relatively wider in the labial-lingual direction near the neck due to the pronounced (lingual) cingulum. The cervical line presents soft convexity towards incisal. The distal face has a uniform convex aspect from the incisal edge to the neck. As the incisal edge slopes upwards towards the distal, the distal face is shorter than the mesial. The root is single, rounded and tapering towards the apex. It is longer in proportion to the length of the crown than in the central permanent. The apical third curves towards vestibular and distal.

■   **Upper lateral incisor**

The upper lateral incisor is situated distal to the upper central incisor and mesial to the upper canine. It is smaller than the maxillary central incisor and less symmetrical. The mesio-distal dimension of the crown is smaller than the cervico-incisal dimension, i.e., the crown is longer than wide.

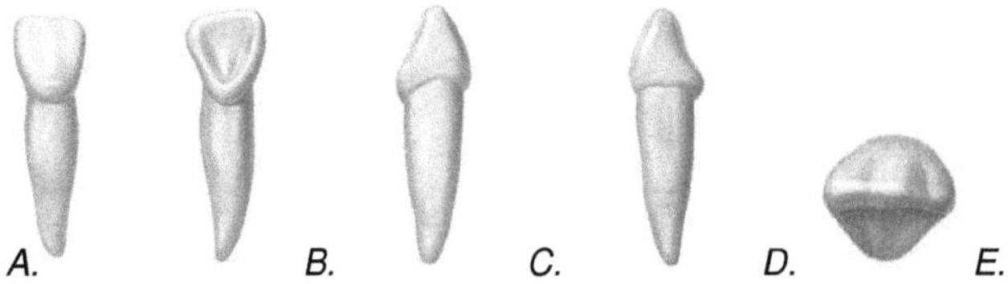

Figure 5 - A. Vestibular face; B. Lingual face; C. Mesial face; D. Distal face; E. Occlusal face.

From the incisal view, the greater narrowing of the mesio-distal dimension is reflected in a more rhomboid and convex contour. The incisal edge is more distally and cervically inclined than the central incisor. The disto-incisal angle of the crown is also more rounded. The buccal aspect of the crown, although slightly convex, is quite flat when compared to the deciduous upper central incisor. It has the largest cervico-incisal dimension than the mesio-distal one. The marginal ridges of the lingual surface are more prominent due to the greater depth of the lingual fossa. The mesial and distal surfaces are convex with the mesial surface slightly wider and more convex than the distal one. Root morphology is similar to the central incisor but proportionately longer. It is flat in the mesial-distal direction with a deviation of the apical third towards the buccal and distal sides.

■ **Lower Central Incisor**

The lower central incisor occupies the most mesial part of the lower hemi-arch. It is the smallest and narrowest of all the deciduous incisors. It shows great similarity with the lower lateral deciduous incisor and also with its permanent counterpart. The crown of the lower central deciduous incisor is symmetrical and flattened towards the mesio-distal direction and very elongated towards the cervico-incisal direction. The mesio-distal and buccal-lingual dimensions are similar. In general, it is 1 mm smaller than the maxillary central incisor.

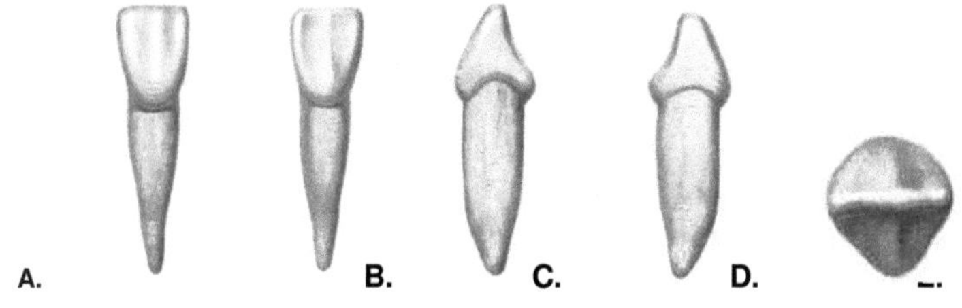

Figure 6 - A. Vestibular face; B. Lingual face; C. Mesial face; D. Distal face; E. Occlusal face.

The incisal edge is straight and thin and divides the crown into two approximately equal halves: vestibular and lingual. The incisal edge is devoid of mamelons and the proximal angles are almost straight. The buccal surface is relatively flat and has no depressions, being very elongated in the cervico-incisal direction. It is slightly convex in all directions, with a protrusion in the cervical portion. This face has a trapezoidal shape. The mesial and distal sides are uniformly convex, this convexity being smaller than the one exhibited by maxillary deciduous incisors. The contact area is in the incisal third of the proximal surfaces. On the lingual surface all sides are similar to those described for the buccal surface, but it is narrower. The cingulum is well defined but the marginal ridges are not as developed as in deciduous maxillary incisors. Thus, the central fossa is quite shallow. The proximal faces are triangular and have rounded sides and angles. They are convex and converge lingually. The labial-lingual dimension is relatively large when compared to the permanent inferior central incisor. The cervical line is convex to the crown, being more convex mesially than distally. The root is single, relatively long and tapered, having approximately twice the length of the crown. The buccal and lingual surfaces are convex while the distal and mesial surfaces are flattened, giving a flattened appearance. Its apical third is deviated to the buccal side.

■ **Lower Lateral Incisor**

The lower lateral incisor is located distal to the lower central incisor and mesial to the lower canine. This tooth is similar to the deciduous central incisor, but it has some differences that allow it to be distinguished. The crown is larger in the mesial-distal and cervical-incisal dimensions.

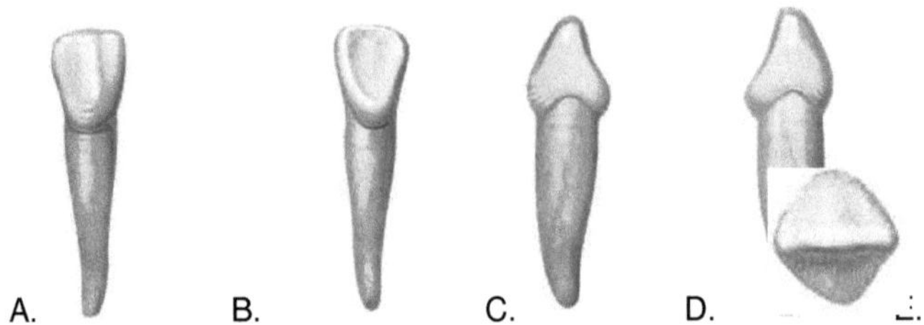

Figure 7 - A. Vestibular face; B. Lingual face; C. Mesial Face; D. Distal Face; E. Occlusal Face.

The incisal edge slopes gently distally and cervically, and the disto-incisal angle is more rounded. The buccal side is very similar to the central incisor, but has larger dimensions. The distal side is a little shorter than the mesial side. On the lingual side the cingulum and the marginal ridges are usually a little more pronounced but the lingual fossa is still shallow. The greater asymmetry of this tooth is evidenced by the distal displacement of the cingulum, as occurs in the lower permanent lateral incisor. The proximal faces are triangular with convex surfaces. As the incisal edge inclines towards the distal and cervical, the distal face is smaller than the mesial face. The root is single, flattened in the mesial-distal direction, and generally has longitudinal grooves. It curves towards the vestibular-distal side, generally in the apical third.

DECIDUOUS CANINE GROUP

■ **Deciduous Upper Canine**

The root of the maxillary deciduous canines is larger than that of the maxillary deciduous incisors. Before resorption, it is the largest root of the deciduous dentition. Moreover, it has a buccal inclination in the apical third and all of it deviates distally. Its mesial and distal surfaces are vaguely leveled. In short, it is wide and tapered. The pulp cavity of deciduous maxillary canines has little demarcation between the root canal and pulp chamber. Like the external contour of other teeth, this cavity is divided into pulp horns, the central, mesial and distal.

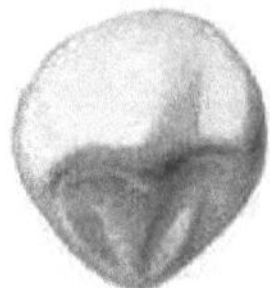

Figure 8 - Incisal view of the upper canine

The crown of these elements reveals a significant narrowing at the neck and is often wider. The buccal-lingual and mesial-distal dimensions are similar. Their incisal edges have a rhomboid aspect with the presence of a well-defined cusp that tapers at its end. On the lingual surface it has a convex shape, its marginal ridges and cingulum are prominent, however, they are not as prominent as in permanent upper canines. There is the presence of two lingual fossae formed by a ridge between the cuspid and the cingulum, these fossae are called mesio-lingual and disto-distal respectively. When observing the buccal surface, more specifically in the cervical third a defined hump that is closely related to the tubercle and Zuckerkandl.

In the mesio-incisal and disto-incisal angles, both are at the same level. However, in terms of width, the mesio-incisal angle is wider than the distal-incisal angle. The cervical side is more concave towards the crown and the cervical line corresponds to that side. The distal side, which is more angulated, has a more rounded structure.

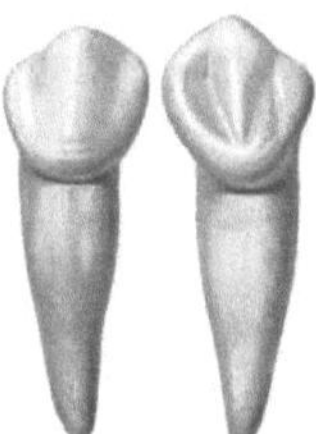

Figure 9 - Buccal and lingual surface of the upper canine

With concave lingual side and convex vestibular side, the proximal faces are convex. Its mesial face is similar to a triangle and has rounded sides. When it comes to the distal face, it diverges from the mesial face in the cervical line, which is prominently more rectilinear.

■ **Deciduous Lower Canine**

The roots of deciduous mandibular canines are smaller than those of deciduous maxillary canines, with a curvature in the middle third towards the vestibular and a slight flattening in the middle distal direction. The pulp cavity does not present differentiation between pulp chamber and root canal, both are thick.

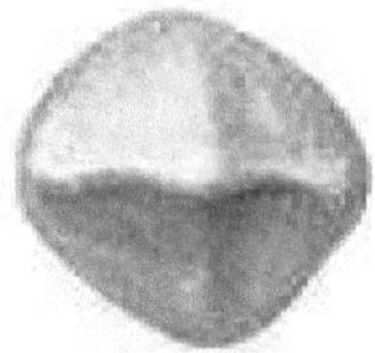

Figure 10 - Buccal and lingual surfaces of the deciduous mandibular canine.

The crown of deciduous mandibular canines is also smaller than the crown of deciduous maxillary canines. Its incisal edge is similar to the upper deciduous canine, differing only in the sizes of the distal-incisal and mesial-incisal aspects, being the distal-incisal larger than the mesial-incisal.

The lingual surface of deciduous mandibular canine teeth has a cervical side, marginal ridge and cingulum which are more imperceptible. Moreover, the buccal surface on its distal-incisal side is wide, consequently, the mesio-incisal side is longer. Moreover, its cusps are pointed and its
cervical line is crooked and concave to the crown.

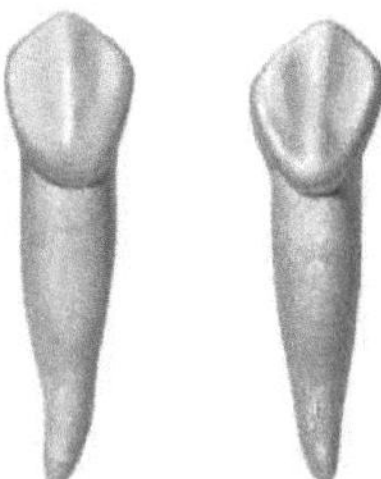

Figure11-Cvestibular and lingual face of the deciduous mandibular canine.

- **First upper deciduous molar**

The roots of the deciduous maxillary first molars are constituted by three divergent and flattened slopes: lingual, distal-vestibular and mesial-vestibular. The lingual is more prominent, longer and wider than the others. Thus, the pulp cavity consists of three root canals respectively the three root slopes, being the lingual root canal longer. The pulp horns are part of the pulp chamber and constitute the cusps.

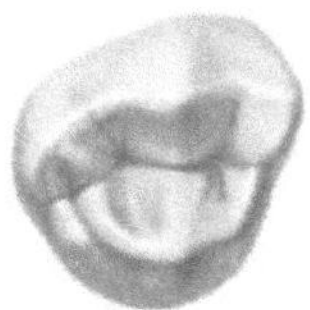

Figure 12 - Occlusal face of the first molar

The crown, in its occlusal view, has rounded angles and a trapezoid shape. Moreover, the occlusal of the deciduous maxillary first molar is shallow and, for this reason, its grooves and cusps are short and superficial. There are the main grooves called mesial-distal and buccal-lingual. The main mesial-distal groove has as function the separation of the lingual and vestibular cusps respectively. The main lingual-lingual groove is not commonly found in the maxillary first molars, it appears sporadically. They are superficial and shallow. The lingual surface does not have grooves and is convex. The cusps are partially seen on this surface. The mesio-lingual cusp is more prominent on the occlusal surface, the distal-lingual and distal-lingual cusps are visible in the lingual view and, finally, the mesio-distal cusp, which has
smaller size.
The proximal surfaces, more specifically the occlusal side of the mesial surface, has a mesial-lingual cusp which is more noticeable and prominent than the others. Moreover, the mesial ridge is short. The cervical side of the mesial face, with the advent of the projection of the buccal boss, presents a larger dimension than the upper permanent molars. The buccal and lingual sides protrude culminally toward the crown, and for this reason, it has a trapezoidal aspect. The distal surface is convex in shape and the contour of the distal-labial cusp is more defined than the others. The buccal surface presents the buccal fossa, called Zuckerkandl tubercle. This face is divided by the main groove vestibular-lingual, constituting the vestibular cusps. The distal and mesial sides also have a convex shape and are well directed to the neck.

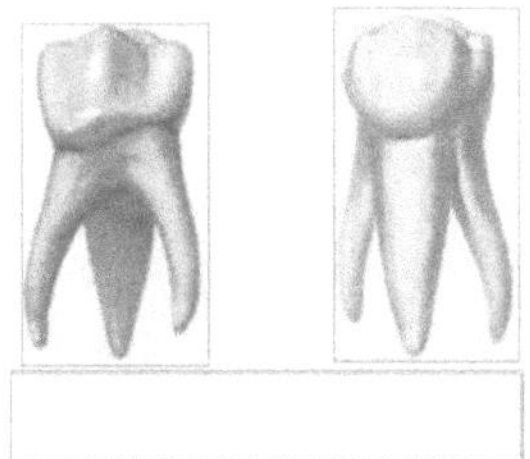

- **First deciduous lower molar**

The roots of the mandibular first molar are positioned in the same way as the permanent mandibular molars. It consists of two roots, one mesial and one distal, are paired in pairs and divergent. Moreover, they are very long and thin, with a strong flattening in the mesio-distal direction. Therefore, the mesial root is always more developed, has a triangular shape and usually contains two confluent root canals at the apex, leaving the pulp cavity between a common orifice. The distal canal, on the other hand, shrinks in the center, although two root canals may also appear in this root.

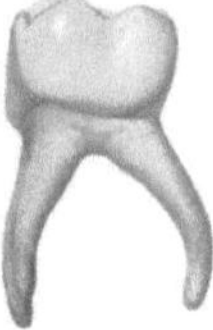

Figure 14 - Lingual face of the deciduous first lower molar.

There is a particularity regarding the crown of the lower first molar, as it does not resemble any other, from deciduous to permanent teeth. Its occlusal surface is slightly ovoid, with a pronounced mesial-distal diameter and four cusps: mesialvestibular, mesial-lingual, distovestibular and disto-lingual. Thus, the two mesial cusps are more noticeable because they are larger than the distal cusps, moreover, they are very proximal and can even be connected by a ridge.

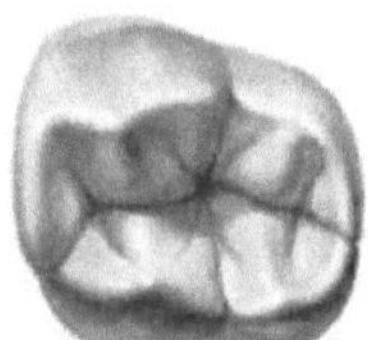

Figure 15 - Occlusal face of the deciduous mandibular first molar.

Still on the occlusal surface, the presence of three well marked fossae can be observed and they have two main grooves: the mesial-distal groove, considered the deepest, which separates the buccal from the lingual cusps and the buccolingual groove which separates the mesial from the distal cusps, besides crossing the mesial-distal groove near the distal extremity of this groove. On the buccal surface the contour of the cusps is more prominent than in the deciduous maxillary first molars. The occlusal side marks the contour of the buccal cusps making the mesiobuccal more evident as it is wider than the distal buccal one. As for the crown, it gains a more intense concavity in the mesial position on the cervical side, besides, the vestibular side in the mesial direction is longer and straighter than the distal side. The lingual side is convex but without depressions or ridges and is shorter in the cervico-occlusal direction than the buccal side. It is composed of two lingual cusps, with the mid-lingual cusp being more broad and tapered. The cervical side is practically straight, while the mesial and distal sides are similar to the buccal side and part of the buccal cusps can be observed from this view. The proximal faces present an irregular trapezoidal shape and have convexities. The mesial surface is larger and flatter than the distal one, with convexity in the vertical third due to the buccal boss and a well-developed mesial marginal ridge. Moreover, its cervical side has different levels and spreads towards the root on the labial side. On the distal surface all four cusps can be observed, but the mesiobuccal cusp is more evident because it is the highest. This face has the characteristic of being convex in all directions and its cervical side is relatively straight since it is located at the same level in the lingual and vestibular surfaces.

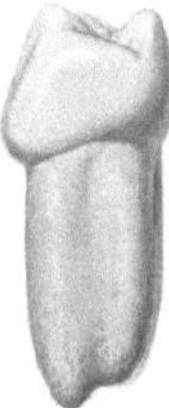

Figure 16 - Mesial face of the deciduous first lower molar.

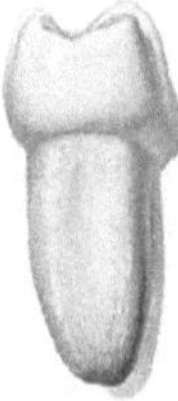

Figure 17 - Distal face of the deciduous first lower molar.

About the pulp cavity, it is worth noting that this tooth has three pulp canals, namely: the distal, which is the largest, the mesiovestibular and mesio-lingual. It also contains a pulp chamber in rhomboid shape.

- **Second upper deciduous molar**

Although the maxillary deciduous second molar retains a similarity in the number of roots with the deciduous first molar, its roots are longer and more hollowed, as well as its crown becomes wider. The root length of the second molar varies between 16.5-18.5 mm. It has three roots, two vestibular and one lingual. In terms of size, the lingual root is the largest, while the distalvestibular root is the smallest among them. Furthermore, frequently the palatal and distobuccal roots are partially or totally united. It also has the potential of four to three independent canals.

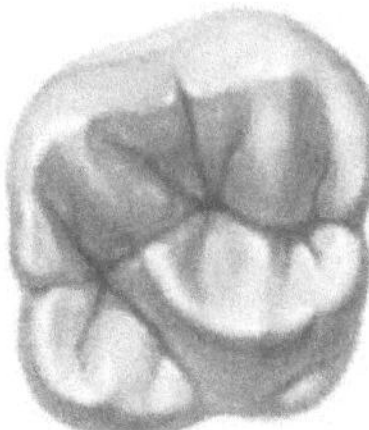

Figure 18 - Occlusal face of the deciduous maxillary second molar.

On the occlusal surface of this tooth, it can be observed the presence of four cusps, and still the possibility of the existence of a fifth. These cusps are well developed and can be described in descending order of size: mesio-lingual, mesio-vestibular, disto-vestibular and disto-lingual. There is still the presence of grooves, pits and ridges. The deciduous maxillary second molar contains a total of three fossae: mesial, central and distal, being the distal the deepest. Regarding ridges, the oblique one, better known as enamel bridge, is very wide and developed, besides it joins the distobuccal cusp with the mesio-lingual one. The buccal surface is composed of the tubercle of Zuckerkandl, located in the mesiobuccal-cervical trihedral angle. As well as, this face is divided by a buccal groove, separating the mesial and disto-vestibular cusps. The lingual side presents a more convex anatomy and quite inclined towards the vestibular side. There may be the presence of Carabelli tubercle in the mesio-lingual portion, and in its occlusal portion is notable the contour of the mesio-lingual cusp.

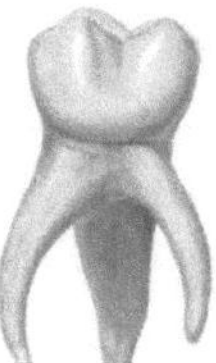

Figure 19 - Vestibular aspect of the maxillary second molar

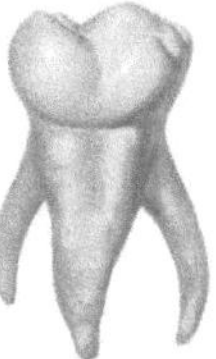

Figure 20 - Lingual face of the maxillary second molar

The anatomy of the proximal surfaces of the deciduous upper second molar can be compared to the shape of an irregular trapezoid, and there is little concavity for the root in the cervical line. The roots are long and divergent. This tooth is triradiculated, i.e., it has two buccal and one lingual root. Another anatomical feature is that the mesial surface is larger and more convex than the distal surface. The pulp cavity is composed of a pulp chamber and three root canals and has four pulpal horns.

■ Second deciduous lower molar

Finally, the deciduous mandibular second molar has a root conformation similar to that of permanent teeth because they have distinct mesial and distal roots. The roots are twice as large as the crown, triangular, long and flattened mesially and distally. Frequently, three canals can be observed, being its distribution two in the mesial and one in the distal, or there can be the presence of only two canals. This tooth has anatomical features very similar to the lower first permanent molar, but there are still some distinctions. Its crown is smaller and its occlusal surface is somewhat reduced than that of the lower first permanent molar. On the occlusal surface, it can be observed the existence of five cusps: mesio-lingual, mesio-vestibular, disto- lingual, center-vestibular and disto-vestibular, described in descending order of size. As well as, it presents three fossae: the mesial, the central being the deepest, and distal with minor characteristic. And its groove system is practically identical to that of the first permanent lower molar.

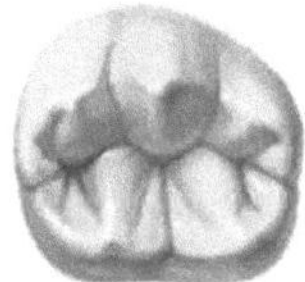

Figure 21 - Occlusal face of the deciduous second lower molar.

The buccal surface is separated by two buccal grooves and can be observed the contour of three cusps, the mesiobuccal, vestibular-center and distobuccal. Another anatomical feature present on this side is the Zuckerkand tubercle, found in the region of the mesio-vestibulo-cervical angle. The lingual surface, in turn, presents a more convex anatomy, and on its occlusal side is observed the contour of the mesio-lingual and disto-lingual cusps, which are separated by a lingual groove. The proximal surfaces of this tooth have the shape of an irregular trapezoid, being the distal surface more convex and smaller than the mesial surface. They contain two roots, one mesial and one distal, they are long, tapered, divergent, flattened and are excavated on the interarticular surfaces because they are responsible for housing the germ of the mandibular second premolar.

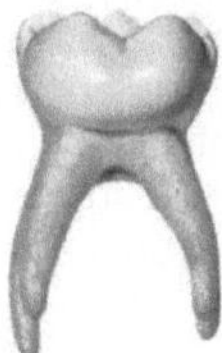

Figure 22 - Buccal aspect of the deciduous second lower molar.

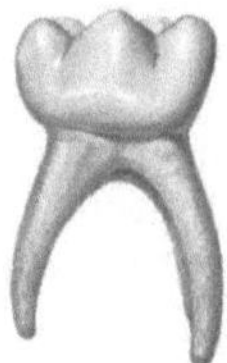

Figure 23 - Lingual face of the deciduous second lower molar.

REFERENCES

MADEIRA, M.C. **Anatomy of the tooth**. 5ª Ed. São Paulo. Editora Savier, 2010.
TEXEIRA, L.M.S.; REHER, P.; REHER, V.G.S. **Anatomy applied to Dentistry**. 2nd
Ed. Rio de Janeiro, 2008.
SAM, **Atlas of Dental Anatomy.**

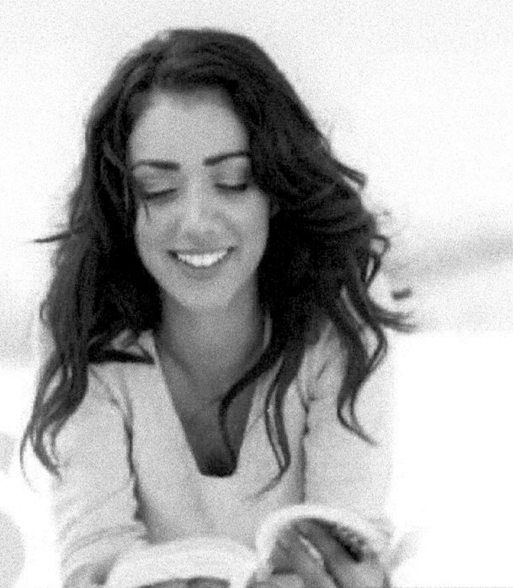

yes
I want morebooks!

Buy your books fast and straightforward online - at one of world's fastest growing online book stores! Environmentally sound due to Print-on-Demand technologies.

Buy your books online at
www.morebooks.shop

Kaufen Sie Ihre Bücher schnell und unkompliziert online – auf einer der am schnellsten wachsenden Buchhandelsplattformen weltweit! Dank Print-On-Demand umwelt- und ressourcenschonend produziert.

Bücher schneller online kaufen
www.morebooks.shop

KS OmniScriptum Publishing
Brivibas gatve 197
LV-1039 Riga, Latvia
Telefax: +371 686 204 55

info@omniscriptum.com
www.omniscriptum.com

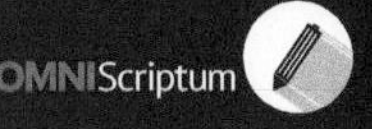

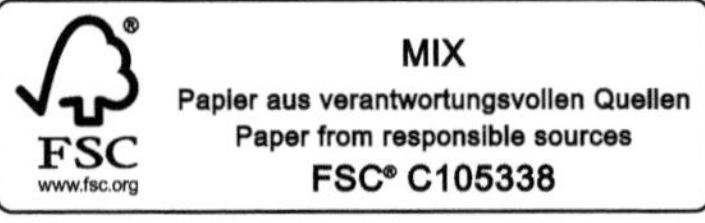

Printed by Books on Demand GmbH, Norderstedt / Germany